FROM MEDROOMS TO BOARDROOMS

Copyright Notice

FROM MEDROOMS TO BOARDROOMS

Copyright © 2017 Hermanuella Hyppolite, RN, CARN, MSN, PMHNP-BC

All rights reserved, including the right to reproduce this book or portion thereof in any form whatsoever.

This book is designed to provide accurate and authoritative information regarding the subject matter covered. It is sold with the understanding that there is not a professional consulting engagement. If legal or other expert advice or assistance is required, please seek a licensed professional in your area.

For information on bulk orders or to have Hermanuella speak at your event, contact Nphyppolite@iberementalhealth.com

DEDICATION

Dedicated to my mother Guyrlene Dorat-Hyppolite, my sisters Beatrice Hyppolite and Isabelle Rachel Hyppolite and my dear friend and mentor Seth Barrington Dressekie - all whom have inspired and motivated me more than they will ever know.

Table of Contents:

Hermanuella Hyppolite, RN, CARN, MSN, PMHNP-BC
FROM MEDROOMS TO BOARDROOMS 6

Arleigh Hatcher, RN ....
SHIFT: FROM BURNOUT TO BOSS 22

Lakesha Reed-Curtis, MSN, RN ....
ALWAYS ON DUTY 37

Brandi M. London, MSN, RN ....
HUSTLE SOLD SEPARATELY: TRANSITIONING FROM
BEDSIDE TO BOSS 50

Dr. Jesslyn Anderson, FNP-C ....
BEYOND THE BEDSIDE 68

Portia "Revlon" Wofford ....
LIPSTICK AND STETHOSCOPES 84

Nicole Tyson-Ferguson, BSN, RN, CM/DN ....
STEPPING INTO MY SEASON 101

Audrey Lovings-Clark, BSN, RN ....
CENTERED BEAUTY: NEVER STOP DREAMING 120

Freda Watson..
> EMPIRE STATE OF MIND 131

By: Drumeka Rollerson, BSN, RN.......................................
> BEDSIDE TO BOSSTRESS 147

Tamara Alford Neely, Medical Director NP-C, MSN, BSN, RN, MT ....
> THE NURSEPRAYNEUR: FROM CARE PLANS TO BUSINESS PLANS 163

Latosha Annan, MSN, RN, DNS-C, CM/DN ....
> NOT YOUR AVERAGE NURSE 181
> References: 200

FROM MEDROOMS TO BOARDROOMS

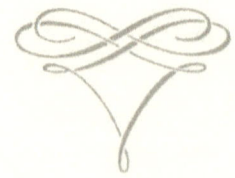

Hermanuella Hyppolite, RN, CARN, MSN, PMHNP-BC

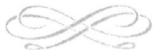

When asked why I chose nursing, I often respond that nursing chose me. I worked my way from an EMT to an RN, BSN, Masters in Nursing/Psychiatric Nurse Practitioner, recently opened my private practice, and am currently working on obtaining my Doctorate in Nursing. I want to share the story of my journey through my nursing career. It has been a journey filled with passion, tears, and hope. I am originally from Port-au-Prince, Haiti; and as far back as I can remember, I have had an interest in health and healing. I remember when I was five years old, a neighbor sustained a burn to her right arm while playing. Just as I observed my grandmother doing so many times before, I took it upon myself to gather some leaves, wash her arms and applied the leaves to the wound using an old shirt. Needless to say, it did not turn out well. At that time, it never dawned on me that my grandmother used a specific leaf for each injury or to even wash the leaves before applying them. My friend's arm became infected, and she had to be taken to the hospital for antibiotic treatments.

I later migrated to the US and, like many immigrants, found difficulty in assimilation when it came to culture and language. I attended Hillcrest High school in Queens, NY, which had an excellent health careers department. Students in the health career track had the option of studying medical assistant, EMT, childcare, or nursing. Those who completed all coursework were awarded a certificate in their chosen track along with their high school diploma. Being young and seeking a thrill, I picked EMT. At 17 years old, I was armed with my EMT-B certificate and ready to conquer the world. I loved the thrill and rush that came with dealing with emergencies. There was just one problem; I was in New York and hated being out in inclement weather. After one year, I started considering other avenues which would allow me to help others and provide the rush that comes with helping someone truly dependent on you. Nursing is such a broad field that I knew I could find a niche which would allow me to utilize my interest in science and the natural world as well as my desire to help people in need. So, in the fall of 2004, I applied to nursing school and started the rigorous two-year program at St. Vincent's School of Nursing in Fresh Meadows NY, all while still working as an EMT. Becoming a nurse is more than just taking a few classes, earning credits, and receiving a degree. When I decided to become a Nurse, I really did not understand the many facets of a Nursing career; I just knew I loved science and I wanted to help people.

Once I did some research and realized how many types of Nursing opportunities existed, I was certain this was the field for me. Nursing is both science and art; memorizing medical facts and procedures are a huge part of the profession, but they can only get you so far. Changing a dressing, inserting an IV, and administering medication does not seem as straightforward when looking into the eyes of patients who at that very moment may be having the worst day of their lives. Halfway through the Associate's program, those who qualified could sit for the Licensed Practical Nurse exam (LPN). After taking and passing on the first try, I decided to take a part-time position at a nearby nursing home and left the ambulance behind. If you have ever been in a nursing home, you know they can be very depressing. Some days I would leave there exhausted and just down right sad. I remember staring at old black and white photos on the walls of the residents that I cared for – pictures of their almost forgotten past. Then, I would look into their eyes and try to imagine all of the life they had lived and seen over the years. I remember thinking to myself many times, "these people I am putting to bed were babies once. Someone loved them and laid them in a crib at night; and now here I am laying them down in their small room with the black and white photos on the wall".

This memory still brings tears to my eyes; it made me sad. I desperately wanted to help them, just talk to them about their lives, and learn from them; but so many of them were "gone" - robbed of their ability to communicate. One day I cared for a woman with ALS (Amyotrophic Lateral Sclerosis) who was bedridden and could only use her eyes and toes. She was still able to operate a computer by using a modified mouse pad and her toes. We communicated via a letter board. Her name was Sarah; I will never forget her. I cry as I write this because she really had a major impact on my choice to pursue nursing as my career. Her walls were covered in photos - not all in black and white, but a few of them in color. She was not old, but the disease had robbed her of many years of her life.

It was frustrating for her not to not have the ability to even scratch an itch. Some days she was in such an awful mood that many of my co-workers refused to work with her, so I would usually volunteer to be her aide. At times, she was so uncooperative that she would stop communicating with me via her letter board. It did not bother me when she was in a bad mood though. It was very easy to empathize with her given her physical state. Her anger was never truly towards me. Sometimes we would just sit in silence in her room staring at the pictures taped up on her wall. It turned out that she had three daughters all of whom lived in different states. She also had grandchildren whom she had never even met because her daughters did not have enough money to travel for a visit with all three. Her son looked like Elvis, and it always made her eyes smile when I would tell her that; so, I said it often. It made her happy, and that made me happy. Working at the nursing home was rigorous, but my love for nursing blossomed even more because it allowed me to realize the impact that I could have on those that I cared for.

A year later, after graduating and passing my state boards exam, I began working at a local private institution on a medical-surgical floor. Many nurses can recall the exact moment in their careers when everything changed - that defining moment when they moved from being a student of the sciences to a master of art behind nursing. For me, this defining moment came soon after I started my career as a Registered Nurse and experienced my first loss. His name was Arthur. He had been suffering with pancreatic cancer for a long time now. Being the new nurse and lowest (wo)man on the totem pole, I usually ended up with the most severe cases. Arthur was bed-bound, incontinent, and required total care and assistance when it came to bathing and eating. Nevertheless, my summer was spent listening to stories about his youth and how much better the sixties were compared to today. And as quickly as the summer passed, so did Arthur. I remember feeling that loss to my core. I had become very close to the family and right after the code, I fell apart. I remember locking myself in the cleaning utility room to cry for close to an hour.

My supervisor at that time was appalled, yelled at me for not being able to hold it together, and sent me back on the floor to finish my shift. I remember going home asking myself, "Was this what I wanted to do for the rest of my life?" When I returned to work that following Monday, my patient's family had witnessed the degrading manner my manager had spoken to me after the code and took it upon themselves to write a letter to the nursing administration. In the letter, they described the compassionate care they had witnessed me providing to their loved one during his last few days. Day in and day out, I cared for him; and still took the time to talk to him as I provided his care. After reading their heartfelt letter, I regained my drive and passion for nursing. Although I cannot save everyone, sometimes all it takes is a back rub, a smile, and a brief conversation about something or absolutely nothing to bring the art of caring back into your work and make a tremendous difference in the lives of those in our care.

Two years after completing my Associates, I decided to return for my Bachelors. It was at this point I started to struggle academically. I don't know what it was, but I felt like I was always fighting an uphill battle trying to catch up with the class material and keep up with my classmates. My anxiety level, especially before exams, increased exponentially and I had to use OTC sleep aids just to fall asleep. It goes without saying feelings of devastation and despair took over. I won't romanticize my feelings at that time and say I knew nursing was for me. Honestly, I felt like giving up; however, I knew I didn't want the past three years to go to waste. What made matters worse is during this time, the facility I worked for went bankrupt and I was forced to find a new job at a new facility and adjust to a new routine and new personalities.

I started working at a local public facility in the Department of Psychiatry. The first few years were rough. The way things were managed in the private sector was not quite the same as the public. Even the patient population differed. Located in the inner city, we catered to more patients of all races and backgrounds, both insured and underinsured. Most of these patients came here because they had nowhere else to go. Nurse-patient ratios were unparalleled to what I was accustomed to at my previous place of employment. I often left work exhausted and unable to do anything else but collapse in bed. No amount of training could adequately prepare me for my first interaction with a psychotic and aggressive patient – a young man, age 21, who had recently suffered from his first break with schizophrenia. The family was devastated and had difficulty accepting that their soft-spoken, shy, intelligent boy who was on a full scholarship to study bioengineering, was now convinced that the family was trying to poison him. Day in and day out I watched as his family brought him clothes and food, but he refused to accept because of this delusion.

On his third week of admission and in the middle of my shift, I observed him wearing a new shirt. When he told me that his brother had given it to him, it was the best news I received that day. It was the first sign that the medications had started to work, and I would soon get to meet the young man that his mother spoke about. My decision to continue with a nursing career was not solidified until I met this young man, the one in the pictures that his mother brought to the unit that looked nothing like the patient I had cared for during the past three weeks. The young man in the picture had a shy smile and barely made eye contact with the camera lens – the total opposite of the one that I cared for who was unshaven, malodorous, and guarded with a fix suspicious stare. He gradually transformed back to the young man the family had been searching for. He soon became a very smart, well-mannered young man with kind eyes. It was at that moment I discovered my niche in Nursing Psychiatry.

According to the Agency for Health Care Research and Quality, in 2004 there were 1.8 million admissions for mental health and substance abuse issues. Often these clients are the sickest as they are unable to care for themselves or have enough insight to seek care when they are sick; however, because of their mental illness and the stigmas associated with working in the field, most nurses prefer not to deal with this population. I, on the other hand, fell in love. I always knew I wanted to work in the medical field and help others; but if you had asked that 17-year-old girl on the first day of nursing school what kind of nurse she was going to be, I would have proudly responded pediatrics of course. Boy, was I wrong! I loved watching the patients transform gradually back to who they were meant to be; and for those who were too ill to return, I occasionally caught a glimpse of their former selves.

Five years into my nursing career, I was commissioned into the U.S. Army as a first lieutenant. Life as an Army Nurse is quite different than that of a civilian, and not just because of the prestige and privileges associated with being a commissioned officer in the U.S. Army. Here, you'll discover unequaled learning and growth opportunities while working in a true team environment and enjoy much more autonomy than what is normally found in the civilian world. The army molds and forces the warrior out of everyone. Being placed in uncomfortable situations such as long hours in the heat, waking up at the crack of dawn, and being forced to push your body to its limit every day causes you to become stronger; and you're able to shrug off things now that in the past may have ruined your day. The army also introduced me to other professionals who have served as mentors and enriched my career like no other. From physicians to social workers, it was a rewarding experience to collaborate and gain a sense of belonging. The army provided me with a second family I will forever be grateful to as they are responsible for me taking the leap of faith by continuing my education, getting my Master's in Nursing/Psychiatric Nurse Practitioner, and recently opening my private practice.

Being an entrepreneur had always crossed my mind, but for years I could not think of a way to start. Becoming a Psychiatric Nurse Practitioner afforded me that opportunity. I am happy to tell you that, today, I have become successful in my career and have currently opened my own practice providing mental health services, medication management, and counseling for individuals across the life span. More and more nurses are breaking free from the bureaucracy of healthcare settings and branching out on their own. I am not just talking about advanced practice nurses; I am talking about the average bedside nurse who wants to see her patients get the care they deserve. This is the nurse who wants to practice the type of professional nursing that makes her feel proud again to be a nurse. The only reason more nurses haven't branched out on their own is because they don't know how. It still surprises me that nurses are not taught how to practice independently under their license and on their own merit and expertise.

Be prepared for the highs and the lows and find ways to get rid of the stress. Keep your priorities in focus. Surround yourself with supportive and positive people. Make sure you have secured the finances and talked to an accountant. For example, it is possible to access your 401K and not have the tax liability if you are investing in your own company. Find an excellent attorney and accountant to protect your assets. Most of all, it is important to be able to take constructive criticism and pivot your business plan when needed.

To be a successful Nurse entrepreneur, you first need to decide on the course you wish to take. What services would you like to offer? Is there a market for those services? If so, who else is offering something similar? With whom can you collaborate? In terms of hard business skills, you must seek the guidance and information you need to formulate a business plan and create your business venture in a guise that works right for you and your specific needs. Ask for help and advice from those who know more than you!

As a new entrepreneur, it is also important to assess your level of risk aversion. Are you willing to quit your job and throw everything into your new endeavor? Or perhaps you're the type of person who would rather continue working a regular job — either part time or full time — and slowly grow your business over time. Either approach has its benefits and detracting elements; it's up to you to make an informed decision based on your particular comfort level.

Finally, make sure you choose an entrepreneurial venture which will be fun, exciting, and interesting for you. Going into business should make you happy, enriching your life on a variety of levels. To be a successful nurse entrepreneur takes time, patience, and consistency. There are many different avenues a nurse can pursue while continuing to work within the scope of her practice. If you intend to diversify and become a nurse entrepreneur, here are few ideas with which to start:

CHILD CARE CENTER

You care for children during the day while their parents are at work or otherwise occupied. You can start a daycare center right in your own home. You will need to purchase small chairs, a table, toys, games, and outdoor play items. Maybe you already have majority of this stuff because you have small children of your own. There are about 75,000 licensed daycare centers in the United States. The price charged for each child ranges from $45 to $200 a week. You'll only need half a dozen kids to make this a high-profit venture.

Most states require a license to run a daycare center. There are several steps involved in getting a license. Call your local State Department of Health and Human Resources to determine the correct office that regulates child care in your state. Call that office and ask for a copy of regulations governing child care centers. Arrange a meeting with a licensing specialist to review the procedures to obtain your license.

NURSE EDUCATOR

Nurses are educated to be health and wellness advocates. The profession is all about restoring optimum health for their clients. Nurses are also taught to be educators. Patient education is about 80% of the job if the job is done correctly. Unfortunately, in the typical acute care setting, nurses do not have the time to do the amount of teaching patients need. Outside of the hospital setting, many opportunities exist for nurse educators. An example would be opening a Home Health Aide school or a program which provides tutoring or exam prep for future nurses.

CONCIERGE NURSE

If you are business minded, a nurse who makes house calls may be the business opportunity for you. In fact, this is historically how most nurses practiced until the 1940s. This area has a huge growth potential. When you start any nursing business, be sure to consult your State Board of Nursing, obtain the proper business and nurse liability insurance, and consult the required experts such as attorneys and tax/accounting professionals. Build a network for up-to-the-minute patient care. With concierge medicine, medical personnel affiliate themselves with a service which charges a group of patients annual membership for house calls and easily scheduled, often same-day, appointments.

PRIVATE NURSING SERVICE

You can establish your private nursing facility where you take care of patients who are undergoing treatment for diseases and injuries. Rather than visit the hospital too often, patients would prefer paying you to study their recovery, dress their wounds, and so on. One mistake you must avoid in this business is assuming the responsibilities of a doctor, especially when you are a nurse or you lack experience on the case at hand. You will maintain your integrity by referring patients to qualified physicians whenever the need arises.

HEALTH BLOGGING

It is interesting to note there are loads of people who are making millions annually through blogging. If you have a medical professional or are someone who has sound knowledge in the healthcare sector, one of the businesses you could consider starting is to blog on healthcare related subjects. The truth is, if your blog has useful and helpful contents, you will attract loads of traffic. If you have loads of traffic on your blog, you can easily secure good advertising deals from stakeholders and other businesses for your blog. Just ensure your blog is updated regularly and you will continue to attract traffic.

Becoming a nurse entrepreneur was the easy part; I woke up one morning and said, "I'm going to be a nurse entrepreneur." It's what follows those words that leads to your success. The first lesson I learned is to not expect things to happen as you planned. In order to be a successful nurse entrepreneur, stay passionate and focused on your dream; listen more; talk less; and learn as much as you can.

Don't second-guess yourself; if you have to continuously ask yourself if you made the right decision to become a nurse entrepreneur, then you're not ready. Confidence is a must because everyone is not going to be as excited about your dream as you, and things are not going to happen overnight. Don't let that make you second guess yourself. Honesty, passion, patience, and respect for yourself and others are things you need to be a successful entrepreneur. What does it take to be a successful nurse entrepreneur? Persistence! Failure is not an option. Stick to your passion and whatever you have experience in to back it up. If you chose the path of private practice on the road to entrepreneurship, keep your eye open for my upcoming guide to Nurse Practitioners opening private practices in New York.

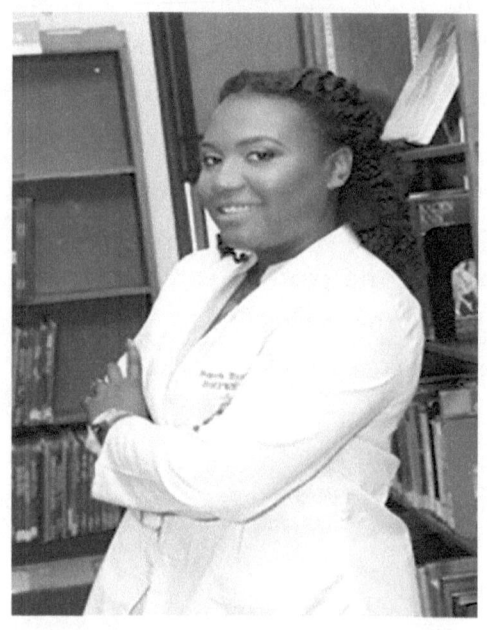

About the Author

Hermanuella Hyppolite, RN, CARN, MSN, PMHNP-BC has been an RN for more than 12 years. Ms. Hyppolite also served in the United States Army Reserves as an Army Nurse Corps Officer in Combat Operational Stress Command (COSC). She received her AS in Nursing at St. Vincent's School of Nursing, and her BSN and MSN at Molloy College. She is certified in Addiction Nursing and is board certified as a Psychiatric Nurse Practitioner. She is currently the Director of the Statewide Peer Assistance for Nurses (SPAN) program by the New York State Nurses Association (NYSNA). SPAN is the confidential education, support and advocacy program for nurses licensed in New York State dealing with or seeking education on substance use disorders. She is also the CEO and owner of Ibere, an outpatient mental health clinic in New York. In her free time, she enjoys traveling cooking and spending time with her family and friends

To Contact The Author:

Ibere, LLC

70 East Sunrise Highway suite 500

Valleystream, NY 11581

Tel: 516-323-8555

Fax: 972-251-6878

Nphyppolite@iberementalhealth.com

SHIFT:
FROM BURNOUT TO BOSS

Arleigh Hatcher, RN

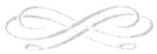

I decided to become an entrepreneur after I became pregnant with my first child. I was working as a traveling Registered Nurse, and I needed to make some big decisions fast! My pregnancy started out real cute at first. My only side effect was being sleepy; I was still cute, and everybody was so happy for us. Then, the sickness started - constant nausea, vomiting, and many other fun activities that come with pregnancy. Being so ill caused me to miss time from work in addition to causing my income to decrease drastically, and that was just not going to work for me. On top of that, my travel nurse status did not allow me to accrue paid leave time, so I had to worry about how long my husband and I could afford for me to be out of work after I had our precious baby girl. That time in my life was when I knew there was so much more I could be doing to bring in a steady income while still having free time for my growing family.

It was then that I knew it was time to make a major shift in my career. I began to research ways I could become my own boss, but I had some hard criteria to fulfill. I knew that whatever the eventual plan would be, it had to please God, serve the community, and somehow incorporate my nursing background. I knew I didn't want to be the mom who worked all the time and never saw her kids. I also didn't want to struggle financially either. The first action I took to figure out my next step was to pick up a book like the one you are reading right now. It was a series of stories about nurses who had taken a leap of faith to start their businesses on their own. There were people who founded home care agencies, travel agencies, CPR training companies, consulting companies, and much more. I was amazed at their courage and I felt that, if they could do it, surely, I could too.

I knew that at first, I could only pursue my business dreams on a part-time basis. I was not ready to let go of my job, so I decided to establish a business that could start off as part-time and eventually get much larger. The very next day, as I was browsing through the course offerings from my hospital, a CPR instructor course popped up; all I had to do was sign up and order the books. That was such a blessing, and the timing could not have worked out any better. I am a firm believer that God puts you right where you need to be, right when you need to be there. Who knew that my path to full-time entrepreneurship would start with a $30 investment back in 2009?!

As soon as I completed the two-day course, I was ready to get started on my new adventure. The first thing I did was get my business license from my local court house. Since it was a home-based business, I just used my county of residence. The process was very easy and not expensive at all. I would advise you to research what kind of business structure will work best for your business, so you can avoid some of the challenges I had when your revenue starts to increase. My next step was to find a website template company who would allow me to build a professional website that fit my business budget. I ended up building my site for $9.99/month, and I added the extra feature that placed me higher in local google searches for an extra $5/month. Keep in mind, this was back in 2009 when I had zero experience at doing anything I was planning to do.

Thankfully, our reliable internet gave me the tools I needed to project a professional and experienced online brand.

At first, my business was subtle and not busy at all. In my entire first year, I only made $5,000 in profit teaching CPR. At the time, I was very proud of that because that money was in addition to my nursing salary; it was generated by my very own business; and I was proud to call myself an entrepreneur with some actual profits no matter how small. For many people, an extra $5,000 is great, heck, for me that was incredible at the time. The problem with the amount was that I was always busy. I was working full time, teaching CPR on all my days off, and spending the rest of my small amount of time with my husband and my then one-year-old daughter. As I mentioned earlier in the book, my goal was to have more time with my family, not less. My limited hours at home was a significant sacrifice for my husband because it left little time for us to connect while I was working to build Heart to Heart CPR. I recall driving for up to an hour just to teach a one-person CPR and First Aide class when I first started. One of the best things I learned in my first year was that my time was just as valuable as the customers' time. It was no longer enough to just be happy that I was making money on my own; I needed to create policies which required a certain number of students before I would travel to their residence. I knew my courses took the same amount of time no matter how many students I had, so I could either make 1x the course fee or 20x the course fee.

For me, time is much more valuable than money, and that is why limit setting is so paramount. Going into my second year, I made sure my website clearly stated that I would only come to business offices with at least five students. Otherwise, they had to come to me. This new policy presented a new problem because I didn't have an office space for them to visit. I was still working entirely from home and traveling to each of my customers individually. The practice of being a solopreneur/mompreneur allowed me to build great relationships with my clients, but it completely stunted my business growth. I was the only employee; I was the web designer, marketer, instructor, manager, budgeter, and much more. The method of doing everything yourself can be necessary when you are first starting out, but you must start your business plan with the end goal in mind. My ultimate goal was always to spend more time with my family without having to sacrifice financially. It was time for me to hire some employees and find a home for Heart to Heart CPR.

Since I worked in a hospital, I had a pool of colleagues to look to as potential employees for my CPR company. I immediately sent out an email and got back a few responses from CPR instructors interested in making some extra money. I still remember how excited and nervous I was to have actual people working for me. I also recall the joy I felt when I was at work one day and had two CPR classes going at one time that were taught by my two new employees. I was beginning to see my dream of leaving my full-time job unfold, but I was still in need of an affordable office space. At the time, I was leery of renting a space since CPR classes would come in waves. It was feast or famine at times for my part-time business, so I had to be cautious to make sure my choices didn't negatively affect my family. While I'm totally down to chase my dreams and take measured risks, my priority will always be my family's security.

I began to comb through office rental listings online; and after a few months, it seemed that nothing appeared to be the right fit for Heart to Heart CPR. I was so close to giving up my dream of becoming a full-time business owner, but then something incredible happened. One day, I was on my way to the grocery store and something guided me to check out a building that was a bit off my route. Keep in mind, I didn't know anybody who rented from this building; I didn't even know if they had space available, something just guided me to check it out. As I went into the building, the building manager happened to be available and showed me a few office spaces. I thought the space was perfect; but when he told me the rental fee, I became terrified and declined on the space. By this time, it was October of 2011, my daughter was two, I was still working full-time, had two employees, and no office space. I decided that maybe I could be ok with my current situation. The employees helped with the CPR classes I would have typically taught on my days off, so I made it ok in my mind for me to put my true dreams to the side. One thing I have learned is just to let God lead the way in all things. I have found that when I force things and stress the most, not much happens; but as soon as I get out of the way, God steps in and shows me that he has a plan for it ALL.

I still can't believe what happened next. December 2011 comes, and I get a phone call from the building manager of the space I loved but declined a few months back. The building manager told me he believed in the service I was offering the community and he wanted to help in any way he could. He said the mission of the building was to do God's work by helping people who want to help people. He then offered me the space for half of the quoted rent and use of all the conference rooms. Perfect for my growing CPR company! I accepted right away and moved in the very next month.

Once I moved in, I quickly found that my business doubled

by just having an office for students to come to. Having an office space worked positively for my service based business. Many successful companies operate from home, depending on their audience; mine just didn't work out that way. As I continued to work full-time and book CPR classes, I began to gain confidence in being an actual business owner. It felt good to be able to contribute to my family and help the community with a lifesaving skill at the same time. I still felt there was something missing.

After about six months in my office, I reached the incredible milestone of working part-time at my job as a Registered Nurse in the hospital. My business was finally beginning to supplement a part of my income, and I was very grateful for that. While I was thankful for the growth, I still felt I could be doing more. Reflecting back, it seems I always feel like I can be doing more, no matter what project I have going on. I started to research other courses I could offer as a Registered Nurse within the community, and I was surprised to find a wide variety of choices. I first started out with adding Medication Aide and Pharmacy Technician Training. Those first two courses created a lot of long nights for me. I was very particular about creating the content required to deliver a quality course. Thankfully, my husband supported me 100% on this journey to be a full-time business owner. While there were times that we disagreed on my newfound obsession with the business, he was ultimately able to understand that this was a temporary situation which would allow our family to have more time together in the future. I was very new to this; but with the help of mentors, Google, and God, I worked it out nicely.

My first Medication Aide class had five students in it, and I was so proud of that. I was able to work even fewer hours at the hospital, only working three days per month, to free up the time to teach my newly approved Medication Aide class. By the time my first Pharmacy Tech course started, I had hired one more employee to teach that class, and we had a flurry of students sign up for the class the very night before it started. My motivation to grow my business was at right around 1,000% by then. I then had four streams of income between my job, Medication Aide courses, CPR training, and Pharmacy Technician training; I was doing pretty well. I was still uncomfortable totally quitting my job, despite finally being able to earn more than I did working in the hospital.

The final push for me to put in my two weeks at work came almost by accident. I had been down to working those three days a month for about four months and toying with sending my resignation letter, but I couldn't gather the courage for some reason. In those months, I added on a Nurse Aide training course which was going to be taught by me Monday-Friday. I was still operating my business with myself, one Pharmacy Tech Instructor, and two CPR instructors. Heart to Heart CPR was beginning to take up most my time, and it was only going to get busier from there. People say that when God wants you to grow, he makes you uncomfortable. Well, I was squirming in my seat, couldn't keep still, pacing the room, sweating missiles nervous. I was completely racked with fears of inadequacy and ultimate failure in my young company. These concerns came mainly from inexperience and an overwhelming feeling of figuring it out as I went along. As I got to know more and more entrepreneurs though, this seems to be a common theme among us all in the very beginning of a new venture. Finally, I took it to God for guidance on how to proceed. I prayed about it and went to bed on it.

Now, I'm not saying that Beyoncé (Yoncé) had anything to do with me finally quitting; but I do know that the next week while watching her HBO special "Life is but a Dream", I was inspired to take that leap from an employee to an employer. I had already been leaning towards putting in my two weeks because the Nurse Aide class that I was starting was rapidly approaching. The only problem was I had zero students, my Medication Aide class had graduated, CPR had slowed down, and if I quit my job prematurely, I feared that I would put my family in a financial bind. On the other hand, what if the class filled up and I earned a bad reputation for not being able to deliver the course for fear of quitting my job. I had some serious choices to make. In the meantime, I decided to draft up a two-week notice to see it on paper and maybe get the guts to send it off. I will never forget on Valentine's Day of 2013, my husband and I were at home because it was on a Thursday and he had to work that night. My daughter was asleep, and I was up watching Yoncé's HBO special sipping a glass of wine. There was this one part where she jumped into the ocean from her yacht and said the most fitting thing for my situation. She said "In my hardest moments, where I thought what am I doing, I'm not strong enough for this, I can't get through this, I'm not ready, I just have to say jump! Because, I know I'm going to land in that water and swim back on the boat and I'm going to jump again and land in the water and swim back to the boat. I have to trust myself." That stuck with me because no matter what happened with my company, I was still a seasoned Registered Nurse at the end of it all and that was enough for me to finally make that "jump." I hit the send button on a notice to my boss, worked my two weeks (at one day per week lol), and I never looked back.

In my first few months without my RN income, it was not easy. My first Nurse Aide class had only two students in it. I decided to run it because one student paid in full and she was so excited to start the class. The other student was sponsored by an agency, and I didn't get paid for two months! It was rough starting out; but with the spiritual and financial support of my husband, mother, and grandparents, I was able to make it through. Some people don't like to talk about receiving monetary help in the beginning, but it is sometimes necessary when your business is just starting out. Just having someone to say, "It's OK, I believe you can make this work" was enough to keep me going many times in the beginning. Thankfully, we gained more scholarship resources, my mentors helped steer me in the right direction, and my company started turning around for the better. There would be no Heart to Heart Career Training Center without the support of my family, and I am so thankful for that.

Taking that leap of faith brought out a better side of me - a more focused, responsible, and understanding aspect to my personality that trained my mind to react with the long-term effects of the situation in mind. Most of my students were young women with children who were doing their best to make it all work. I was 28 years old at this point in my business, juggling my home life with my professional life and, mostly, trying to make it all work myself. My understanding of the difficulty of being a modern woman with children made it natural for me to create lifetime bonds with many of my students. Life can get so hard, and I love being able to help people get to the next level despite difficult circumstances. At the same time though, experience has taught me that being equally firm and fair was an integral part of running a successful company.

Being a nurse business owner has shaped my business by giving me the confidence to reach for the goal of full-time entrepreneurship. Knowing I had the ability to succeed at becoming a Registered Nurse gave me the confidence to start my own business with success as an expectation. I also knew that if for some reason this business didn't work out, I could always go back to being a Registered Nurse in the hospital. Being a nurse has also given me credibility as a business owner even early on when I was in my startup phase and learning many lessons along the way. On the first day of operating my vocational school, nursing gave me years of credentials as an educator because of my experience teaching CPR, giving patient education, and orienting fellow nurses to my unit.

In the four years since I decided to trust my abilities and quit my job, Heart to Heart CPR has become Heart to Heart Career Training Center; we have added Phlebotomy, EKG Technician, Medical Billing and Coding, Online Monitor Technician, and Online Pharmacy Technician as well as a CPR Instructor course to our roster. As I write this, we have just opened a second location in the Northern Neck area of Virginia. After being open for only a week so far, all our classes for that school are nearly filled. I have also transitioned from teaching altogether so I can focus on continuing to grow my company. Praise God!

5 Tips to Shifting from Burnout to Boss

1. Trust the process and understand that how it is right now, isn't how it will always be. Seeing the bigger picture is what has kept me going during the hard times of my business.

Being an entrepreneur comes with the good and the bad, especially during the startup phase.

2. The phrase "Your network is the key to your net worth" is so true. Networking should be consistently done through social media sites, at conferences, and everywhere that you go. Connecting with people and sharing what you do could be the key to get you in the position to reach your full potential as an entrepreneur or on your career journey. I have met the most incredible people through social media, including the Nursepreneurs featured in this book.

3. Protect your energy! Guard your eyes and ears from negativity by filtering what shows up on your social media timelines and in your life in general. Negative energy is fully transferrable in many ways, and at times we may not realize how social media can affect us.; Even though you may not be posting negative things, those things that you see, read, and hear affect your energy and therefore affect your results. I make a conscious effort to be consistently exposed to likeminded people who inspire me and push me to accomplish greater things. It has made a significant difference in my life, and it bring me so much joy to know that on a bad day I can hop online and get an energy boost from what my friends are achieving.

4. Hire people when its time. When I first started, I used to do everything; marketing, web design, social media, office work, answering the phones, teaching classes, everything was my responsibility. At first, I was ok, but I realized that there was no room for me to grow my business if I was constantly working inside the business handling the day to day operations. It took me a few years to get comfortable enough to hire

people to do 90% of the tasks required to run my business. Having a strong team allows me to dedicate time to my family, friends, and other business ventures. For some, it may be fine to be a solopreneur indefinitely, but I always knew I became a business owner to create free time for myself. My first year (or two maybe) in business was filled with 16-hour days and all-nighters; but seven years after starting my first business, I am quite proud to work a regular schedule mostly from home with the ability to show up for every event in which my children are involved. I'm thankful I can be an entrepreneur with the ability to spend quality time with my family.

5. Invest in people who know more than you. Google and Youtube are helpful, but they don't know everything. Hiring a coach has been instrumental in my businesses growth and online presence. There are coaches who specialize in business, branding, finances, automation, and much more. Hiring an expert in an area where you are lacking can take your business to the next level and set your business apart from other companies.

Most importantly, never give up because of a little discomfort; learning to shift is essential to your growth into a true Boss. In business, I have faced many obstacles but never chose to stop nor turn around. The choice to shift has been what has kept me grounded and continuously moving forward even during the hardest times. I encourage the readers of this book to shift when necessary, seek help when needed, and always look for a way to serve others in each endeavor that you take on! It all starts with the Shift!

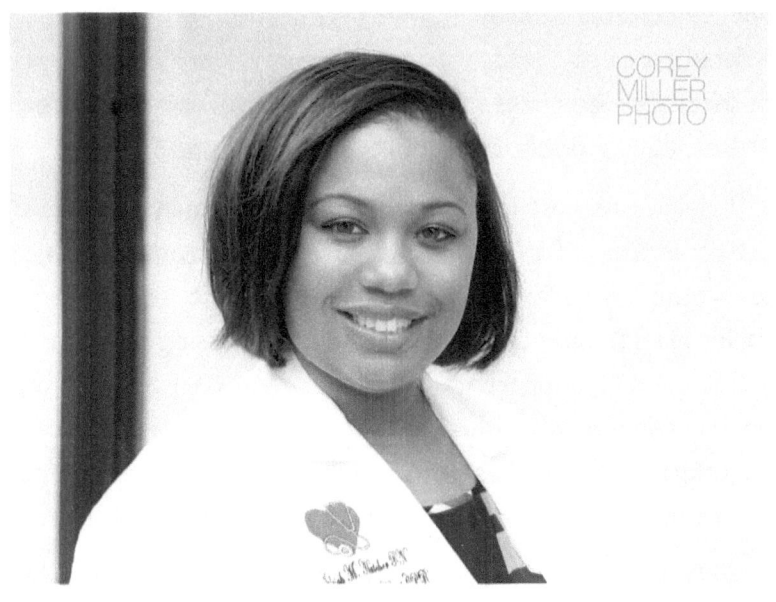

About the Author

Williamsburg, Virginia's own Arleigh Hatcher is a born and raised native of York County and proudly upholds her family legacy of contributing to her local community in many ways. Bred from a deep-rooted history of women who save lives, she followed the family profession of becoming a nurse but has evolved into so much more. As a wife and mother of two, Arleigh touches the lives of people of all backgrounds through her school Heart to Heart Career Training Center as well as her newest family business Peek of Joy 3D Ultrasound & Spa, both based in the city of Williamsburg. Instructing young aspiring professionals as well as experienced and mature students for the past seven years, her influence reaches far beyond the hands she shakes when she bestows upon them their certificates. Through her certification programs, these professionals go into our community, providing quality healthcare for our parents, grandparents, and young children in our hospitals, schools, doctors' offices, and homes.

Arleigh's newest joint venture with her family touches the next generation of Williamsburg natives even from deep within the womb by offering a special experience for expecting families via 3D and 4D imaging. Fusing the classic style from her mother and grandparents with her "new-school" forward thinking, she innovates this corner of the maternity industry by also offering the families who visit their studio and spa many ways to immortalize such a special time-period in their lives.

This wildly successful young entrepreneur has been invited to speak to and inspire other young women who are looking to combine their passion and talents to provide for their families by owning their own businesses. Email admin@hearttoheartctc.com for booking.

To Contact The Author:

Instagram- @theentrepreNurse_, @peekofjoy3d, and @hearttoheartctc

Facebook- Arleigh Hatcher

ALWAYS ON DUTY

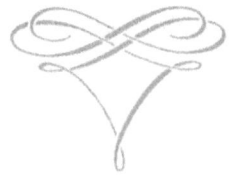

Lakesha Reed-Curtis, MSN, RN

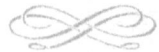

So, you are a nurse and now you want more? I totally get it. I was once in your shoes, wanting more and just trying to figure out a way to live out my dreams. Seven years later, I am doing just that. Let me give you a little information about myself before I dive in. I am Lakesha Reed-Curtis MSN, RN and the President/owner of Allied Health Academy, Medical Solutions Academy, Inc. which was founded in 2011. I also recently started Dream ChasHers, a women's networking group that encourages you to chase your dreams while having other successful women cheering you on. I have an amazing ten-year old son, KeShaun, and a beautiful 1-year old daughter, Madison, and have been married to my adoring husband Terrel for three years. I have been a Registered Nurse for fifteen years and received both my Bachelor and Master degrees in Nursing at Winston-Salem State University.

Now if you want to know why I chose to be a nurse, let me tell you where I received my initial inspiration. I cannot remember my exact age, but I was around eleven or twelve when the idea was brought to me. My cousin Courtney and I were at my grandmother's house and he had a nosebleed, so I ran to his aid. I remember my grandmother saying, "Girl, you should be a nurse." That's right, you know how grandmothers are; any little thing you do right, she cheers you on. She spoke that destiny over my life for the rest of my teenage years; so, when it was time for me to go to college, my major was

Nursing. It's funny how things happen in your life and how you can speak things into existence. Ironically, I don't remember my cousin ever having another nosebleed. Call me crazy, but maybe God allowed that nosebleed to happen at that instant so my grandmother could speak over me. Honestly, if I didn't have that programmed in my head for so many years, I don't know where I would be or what I would be doing. Thanks grandma!!!

When it was time for college, I left home for Old Dominion University and managed to stay for one whole semester. Yep…only one semester. I was extremely homesick and knew the environment wasn't one to which I could adjust to. I came home for Christmas break and never went back, except to retrieve my things. So here I was back at home with my family looking at me crazy, wondering what I was going to do next. I applied at my local community college and was accepted into the Practical Nursing Program. I couldn't afford to go straight into RN school because of the time frame it required. I needed to finish quickly so I could start working in the field. Once accepted, my grandma was very ecstatic. I remember telling her, one day I may open my own school. It was a joke at the time, but look at me now! That is a prime example of projecting your dreams into the universe and seeing them come to fruition. I truly believe that with all my heart. Before you go any further, speak your heart's desires into the atmosphere and watch God work. Keep Him close. That's the first step.

Upon completing the Practical Nursing Program, I practiced as an LPN for three years and moved to Hampton, Virginia to purse my RN degree. I received my Associates degree from a local community college and stayed in Hampton for three years before returning to Danville, Virginia again. I then received my Bachelors from Winston Salem State University. After receiving my Bachelor in Nursing, I eventually moved to Charlotte, North Carolina in hopes of creating more opportunities for my son and I. With this move came a new job opportunity as Assistant Director of Nursing for a company in the Concord area. I was making a pretty decent salary with this company, but I just constantly felt like something was missing. I needed the freedom to live on the edge a little, take business risks, and make my own choices without the constraints of a set schedule or someone else's rules. I don't think people realize how working for someone else consumes your whole life; all areas are dictated by work because of that tight schedule that comes with it. I was sick of asking for paid time off to take vacations, have a "me" day, or even run errands! And let's be honest, thirty minutes is just not enough time to enjoy a nice lunch. I knew I couldn't work a regular nine to five job long-term and I needed to make a change quick!

Starting my own business had always been something I wanted to do, but I was skeptical of my own abilities and the great unknown of self-employment. It was time for me to stop feeling like I was missing the mark and do something about the unsettling feeling that had been haunting me daily. I just had to figure out what my niche was. I knew I wanted to help my community in a different way than what was already being provided. My main objective was to constantly learn and advance in whatever I chose to do with the goal of success as the common denominator. Most importantly, I wanted to be home with KeShaun as much as possible once he started school.

I remember working the job as Assistant Director of

Nursing, living a good life, but all the while realizing this was not enough sustainable income to take care of my baby and I. I mean life was good, don't get me wrong; but I knew it could be better. I needed it to be better. During the years that I worked from nine to five, I found myself deeply craving the ability to spend more time with KeShaun. By the time I picked him up from daycare, it would be dark outside and the day was already over. It was during those times I set a goal to be at home with him daily before he started Kindergarten; at the time, he was only two so I had a little leeway before he started school. I would sit around and just pray for a business idea to come to me, all the while never losing focus or hope in my dreams.

One night as I was lying in bed with KeShaun, the idea of selling scrubs came to me. In that moment, I hugged him so tight and began to jump up and down in the bed! I remember it all so well. I thought big, but started small. I knew my dreams would not allow me to remain small and growth was in my future. I begin doing trade shows at local nursing homes and sold scrubs to most of my co-workers and nursing friends. Little did I know, this was the start of my entrepreneurial journey! My best friend's mother allowed me to have my first trade show at her nursing facility. My best girlfriend would travel with me in my Camry to the facility two hours away, all squished up and surrounded by the scrubs I was carrying up the road to sell. We still laugh about it to this day! I can look back and laugh at it now, but back then this had become my livelihood and my ticket to working for myself. It just goes to show, it doesn't matter how small you start as long as you start somewhere.

I always liked education and knew I would one day go into nursing education; however, I never actually imagined I would be the owner of a school. Selling scrubs was something I did on the side while I worked my full-time job, but the moment that sparked the idea for what would be my life altering business venture was being terminated from my job. As a graduate of nursing school, I quickly recognized that nursing programs were becoming a trend in North Carolina. This piqued my interest since I had always had the desire to teach. I quickly began researching the requirements and qualifications necessary to become a nursing instructor. This turned into me submitting my application not only to teach but also to open my own school! Ironically, I was terminated from my job as Assistant Director of Nursing in November 2010 and Medical Solutions Academy opened in April 2011. Who would have known that I could get the ball rolling within just a five-month time frame? God is amazing! To this day, I wonder if I had not gotten fired would I have been brave enough to quit the job and follow my dream? It's hard for me to say; but at the time my back was against the wall, so I did what I needed to do. I refused to let another individual or company determine the fate of my family. In my eyes, I had no other options so I stepped out on faith and started MSA.

When I was terminated from my job, I was already in the process of submitting my paperwork to the Board of Nursing to have my Nurse Aide program approved. During this time, my life was very stressful. I was in the process of buying a house, I had just lost my job, and my lease was running out on my apartment. The broker of my home was telling me to find another job so I would not lose my house, but I refused. I had faith and was determined God would see me through; however, I did find a part-time job teaching at a local Nurse Aide school. I only worked there for about two months because my program was quickly approved. Not to mention, I had received the approval to move into my new home and had started that process as well.

To move forward with my program, I had to have a building to hold the courses. For some, an obstacle like this would steer them off course; but once again I kept the faith and allowed God to steer me in the right direction. A local realtor allowed me to use the address on my paperwork until I was approved without paying anything. See how God works things out when you choose not to stress and let him lead the way? So as soon as my program was approved with a pending site visit, I literally had one week to set up my school completely. I had been purchasing equipment along the way, so the process was not too strenuous. Now my first building/school was very small. It consisted of three rooms, which were not connected. I painted those rooms my favorite royal blue color and was on my way. I was so proud. I was also thankful to God most of all for seeing this through. My major goal was to be at home with my son daily once he started Kindergarten; but I had the opportunity be home once he started Pre-K which was even sooner than planned. God is amazing!

Once my school opened in Danville, Virginia, I was blessed with a full class from the start. I truly believe this was because I put a little buzz in the community a couple of months before I opened. You know how some people say don't tell others your dreams? Well, I am the opposite. If you know your dreams are going to happen, then tell someone. You don't want to open a business and not have the word out to the public that you are about to open. Word of mouth is always a good marketing tool especially in a tight knit community. Just remember, any time you tell people your dreams, there will always be a few who will try to deter you from following your desired journey; but never let anyone else determine your path in life. You can do whatever you set your mind out to do!

When I initially opened MSA, I had a secretary and worked sixteen hours a day for the first year. I taught the day and evening classes. I was so tired, but it was the most fulfilling thing I had ever done. For once, I really was the BOSS. Now I don't want you to think that being a nursepreneur is all glitz and glamour. It is hard work, but dreams do become a reality if you put in the effort. Despite the time and effort I was putting into teaching these classes, the reward for my work was priceless. Don't get confused and think those times will not come when you have no one to talk to and you are in the closet crying. You know what I mean, the ugly cry. Trust me, you will be broke at times either because business is simply slow or you have just invested a lot of money in your business; but let me tell you this, money should be the least of your worries. You have the money in your brain and you will reap the benefits of your labor sooner than you think. Just get started. Slow progress is better than no progress. You don't want to have any what-ifs lingering in your head.

After the first year of business, I was finally able to hire staff and return to my home in North Carolina. Yep, I opened a business located two hours away from my home in Charlotte back in my hometown. Now this part of my entrepreneur journey is still the hardest to manage. If my staff gets low, I may have to stay away from home for a couple of days. If things go array, I cannot be there in the blink of an eye because I live too far away. I sometimes think about moving closer to my establishment, but that would defeat the purpose of being an entrepreneur. I like the freedom entrepreneurship establishes; therefore, I feel as though I should be able to work from anywhere in the world. But, the thought stills lingers in my head.

Medical Solutions Academy now has a Nurse Aide, Medication Aide, Pharmacy Technician, Medical Office Assistant, Medical Assistant, a CPR course, and a Phlebotomy Technician program. I am currently in the process of obtaining a Practical Nursing Program. Boy oh boy, that process has been long and arduous; I could write an entire book on that task alone. Let's just say some things don't come to you as fast or as smooth as you want them too; but when you keep the faith, they will come to pass.

Although being an entrepreneur has granted me the desired freedom to work as I please, we all know being the boss is not easy! Couple that with being a mom and a wife and you have reached a completely new level of being on demand for your time. Every woman will have her own set of rules and guidelines she lives by to balance her everyday life. My one and only rule is God first, then family, and THEN business. I live by this and try my best to follow this day in and day out. Anytime I tend to stray from this line of order, it seems like my whole world turns upside down. When things tend to go wrong, I check myself to make sure I'm following my golden rule. If I find that I've switched that order, I'll immediately start praying and ask God to align my vision to his again. My purpose in starting my business was given to me through the talents with which God blessed me and He will forever come first in my life. My family is and will always be my main priority on Earth; therefore, although my business is my baby, it will always come third in my life.

Giving up honestly has never been a thought to cross my mind. I do have those moments when I say forget this, I am going to find a job; however, I get over that in 20-30 minutes flat. Who would I be kidding? I am an entrepreneur by nature and at heart. The process does get hard and you will face a lot of adversity. Sometimes it comes from those closest to you. But if God can see you to it, He will see you through it. I have moments when I question myself. Who am I to start a school and have all these big dreams and goals? But as I knock those goals out, I am quickly reminded of who I am... Lakesha Reed-Curtis, a dreamer and a doer. I honestly believe there is nothing I cannot accomplish with God, the right team, and the right mindset. This is something you must remember - nothing great can be done alone and you must pay to play. Don't try to get everything done for free. Words that my husband always tells me are, "You get what you pay for." This is so true. Invest, Invest, Invest in your business! I cannot stress this enough. It is also important to have a good lawyer and accountant in your corner early in business. I wish someone would have told me that before getting started, but this is one of the many lessons I have learned along the way.

I also suggest having multiple streams of income. Medical Solutions Academy is my bread and butter; however, I like to invest in real estate on the side. Renovating properties has become a passion of mine and has allowed extra money to flow into my life so I can have more room to grow Medical Solutions Academy. It is a lot of work, but I love to see a place once deemed unsuitable for living transform into a warm and cozy place for someone to call their home. Just as with MSA, because I enjoy dabbling in real estate and renovating properties, it feels like less of a job and more of a destiny that

God purposefully placed on my path.

You will face many obstacles on your journey to entrepreneurship, but passion will take you where you need to go. When you stay focused and put your all into your dreams, it begins to feel as if your back is against the wall. You will either fold and go back to working for someone else, or you will be driven that much more to continue your pursuit of reaching your goals. No matter how difficult my journey may have gotten, turning back was never an option for me. I had my son depending on me and I was determined to not only be a good mom, but to also be present as much as possible. I already had the passion for nursing; coupled with the desire to be at home with my son as much as possible, these two factors gave me the motivation I needed to see my dreams come to fruition.

If you can control the way your mind thinks of being a nursepreneur, I strongly believe you will make it through the process. Too often we allow self-doubt and fear creep into our minds and gain control of our thoughts. Suddenly, what once seemed easy now seems impossible all because of negative thinking. We are our own biggest enemy in life. Next thing you know, you're convincing yourself not to quit your job and go into business for yourself because it seems illogical. If you focus on what could go wrong instead of all the things that are going right, then everything will fall apart quicker than you could ever imagine. You must have faith in yourself; and on the days you can't put faith in yourself, put it in God because there is absolutely nothing he cannot do. What is meant for you is for you and no one can deter you from receiving your blessings. I am constantly looking for new ways to build my empire and leave a legacy for my family and ALWAYS ON DUTY.

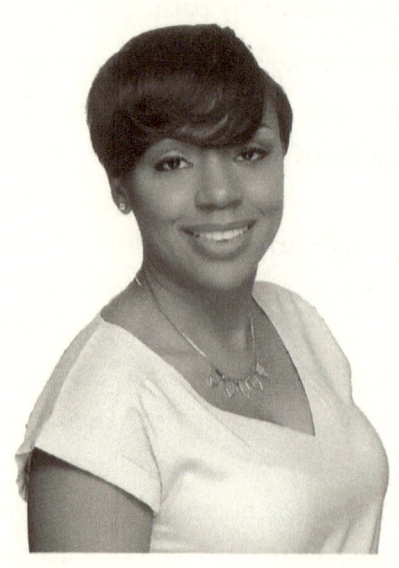

About the Author

Mrs. Lakesha Reed- Curtis, wife and mother of two, is a woman of action who dreams big and just decided to chase hers! She was born and raised in Danville, Virginia, but now currently resides in Charlotte, North Carolina with her loving family. Her focus in life has always been to find different avenues with the opportunity to provide services to the community. Her goal then became to provide higher education opportunities for students interested in the healthcare field to advance career wise in the future. By introducing Medical Solutions Academy to her community, she has become dedicated to empowering her community through educational programs that serve to make prospective health care workers prepared for employment in the medical field.

Lakesha Curtis has fifteen years of hands-on nursing experience and received both her Bachelor and Master degree from Winston-Salem State University. By establishing Medical Solutions Academy, she has gained adequate experience in the full process of operating and administrating successful medical certification programs from start to finish. She has had the opportunity to witness students complete these certification programs over the course of the last seven years. Her educational program has expanded over the years and now includes Nurse Aide, Phlebotomy Technician, Pharmacy Technician, Medical Assistant, Medication Aide, Medical Office Assistant, CPR Certification, and soon LPN. She has built this school from the ground up and enjoys playing such an important role in others' lives.

Constantly facing the demands of maintaining a family and a career simultaneously, Lakesha understood how difficult it is for some women to chase their own dreams. She saw the need to form a group of empowering women to keep each other motivated, which sparked the beginning of Dream ChasHers. She plans to host even more events in the future and build Dream ChasHers into another one of her empires. Although she may wear many titles, she wears them all effectively and efficiently while encouraging other women that they have the power to do the same.

To Contact The Author:

Dreamchashers.com info@dreamchashers.com
Instagram @lakesha_curtis, @dream_chashers, @medicalsolutionsacademy

Facebook: Facebook.com/lakeshareed

LinkedIn: Lakesha Reed-Curtis MSN, RN

HUSTLE SOLD SEPARATELY: TRANSITIONING FROM BEDSIDE TO BOSS

Brandi M. London, MSN, RN

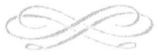

Nursing school was no joke for me. Long hours in the library. Shoulder fatigue from carrying a backpack loaded with twenty-pound textbooks. It was hours reading and re-reading content trying to understand how a disease process affects the body at the cellular level (my medical-surgical professor wore me out with those care plans). My fellow nurses understand my pain and struggle. The journey through nursing school isn't necessarily a bed of roses for anyone. We've all succumbed to the stress in some way or another, right? Either through sleepless nights, mumblings of not-so-pleasant words under our breath as the professor assigned another APA-style paper, or displacing our stress onto loved ones through short temperaments.

You see, I understand the common trials and tribulations shared by nearly every accomplished nurse; but some of our struggles are unique to our own reality. The truth is, nursing school never saw me coming; society never saw me coming; some of my peers never saw me coming. Yet, here I am standing tall. By all accounts, I should've been the least likely candidate for completing college, earning a degree, and earning $60,000 per year in my career by the age of 22. I'm the product of a single-parent home where most of my childhood was spent growing up in public housing or benefiting from public assistance. I was pregnant with my first-born son at the age of 18, giving birth two weeks before my high school graduation. I've suffered through physical and sexual abuse and bouts of depression. Despite it all, I knew there was purpose to my life. So, statistics didn't matter. What society thought was possible was nothing compared to what *I* thought was possible.

My experience in the nursing field spans a variety of clinical settings including telemetry, medical-surgical, progressive care, emergency care, and critical care nursing (just to name a few). Though I love the nursing profession and the amazing opportunities afforded to me due to this profession, nursing was something I sort of stumbled upon. If you were to peruse my high school year book, you'd find a picture of a young, brown-skinned girl with acne-prone skin and tightly-curled bangs. Under that picture, you'd read the caption, "Brandi Walton – Butler University – Pharmacy Major." I received my acceptance letter to Butler University in March 1997, and I was so excited mostly because my assigned roommate was not only a good friend, but she was also family – I was slated to room with my cousin. I don't know what excited me most, the chance to live on my own (sort of) or the chance to get out of Gary, Indiana. Either way, my fate was sealed (or so I thought), and I was on my way to achieving everything I wanted.

We know if we want to make God laugh, we should share the plans WE have for our lives. Well, the plan for my life post-high school changed drastically when I learned during my senior year of high school that I was pregnant with my first-born son. Outside of the shame I felt as a teen mom (though it all worked out as my baby daddy is now my husband), I was even more terrified of how my life would turn out now that I was expecting a child while being a child myself in many aspects. I was terrified of being stuck in the same rut I saw in so many other women in my community who had stories like mine. I was determined to change the trajectory of my life despite the finger-pointers, naysayers, head-shakers and doubters. I even had a nursing professor who had the nerve to tell me she didn't think I could finish the program. I knew education was my only option to make sure the Medicaid, WIC, and TANF lines in which I was standing were only temporary. I finished nursing school in four years and with academic honors. Fifteen years later, I can truly proclaim my love for the nursing profession and my nursing colleagues, particularly for African-American and minority nurses.

The truth of the matter is that none of us are exempt from hardship or struggle while pursuing a goal or dream. I remember clear as day, my dream of obtaining a degree (one of the few women in my family to do so) and creating a life for my family better than the one I knew growing up. It was not an easy road, and the struggles were very real. Once I finally earned my Bachelor's of Science in Nursing, I went on to start a career that quickly changed my perspective of the nursing profession. I expected the work to be challenging, but I never expected to encounter some of the barriers often talked about but rarely addressed in nursing. You know what I mean – nurse bullying and incivility, lack of diversity, and oversight of the contributions of black healthcare professionals in the workplace.

As a black nurse, the struggles are amplified (in my opinion) as it relates to inclusion, representation, and recognition in the nursing profession. In the U.S., only 9.9% of Registered Nurses are black.[i] The Registered Nurse profession is less diverse than the U.S. workforce altogether. A research study conducted in 2013 revealed that nearly 75% of the RN workforce in the U.S. was comprised of white, non-Hispanic individuals.[ii] When we think about minority women in nursing AND business, the inclusion, representation, and recognition are even less.

We understand the negative impact in our communities created by lack of diversity in nursing; this dynamic is part of the reason we celebrate the graduation of fellow black nurses and welcome them with open arms into the profession. The social and professional organizations for black nurses tend to focus on emotional support of those aspiring to enter the profession and those advancing their career through specialty certification and advanced degrees. These accomplishments are incredible and certainly worthy of our recognition and respect; but what are we doing beyond the letters, degrees, and titles to positively impact the profession for our fellow sisters in nursing and those to follow? What are we contributing to the growth of the profession as minority women, leaders, and healthcare providers? Some argue that while diversity in nursing is a growing trend, the African-American presence will continue to lag for some time in the profession. Now, more than ever, we must make our presence felt in our profession. And, we must do this for the sake of our own advancement and for the advancement of those who follow.

For me, I thought my greatest impact would be at the bedside. At the tender age of 22, I graduated with an honors degree and soon after was privileged to put those two big letters behind my name – R.N. I was ecstatic because I was hopeful. I envisioned all the great work I'd do in my community to help my people heal. I remember vividly the picture I painted in my head of one day earning a Nurse Practitioner designation and opening my own clinic (my goals have changed a little since then). Patient care has been a huge component to my career, but I always knew entrepreneurship was for me; not just so I could call myself a boss, but because I always wanted to help others on my terms. As a kid, I didn't dream of fancy weddings, big houses, or fancy cars. Growing up in abuse and lack challenged me to want to help others as much as I wanted to be helped; so, nursing seemed like the perfect fit. The motive for my decision was about more than the letters.

I entered the nursing profession as a hopeless romantic, if you will. In my head, based on a perception that I concocted amongst myself, I romanticized the profession of nursing. I went into it eyes wide shut, with big dreams to change the world by choosing a career path that was all about caring for and serving others. Little did I know, the profession was not as friendly, caring, and loving as I thought. I've learned many things over the years working as a professional nurse. One of the most important lessons I've learned is that we don't make an impact in this world through jobs and titles. Our greatest impact manifests through our desire and willingness to serve beyond ourselves. As I journeyed further into my career, from novice to not-so-novice, I lost track of this very important concept.

For more than 10 years, I worked as a bedside nurse. The first five years were amazing. I started my work in telemetry and found that I absolutely love the heart! I loved working in high-acuity settings with drips, monitors, post-surgical care, observing heart catheterizations – I loved it all. I learned a ton about delegation and time management, and picked up nursing skill sets that made me very marketable as a nurse. My resume boasted work in some of the best facilities in my area – some even recognized nationally and globally as the best in the type of care provided. Before I knew it, seven years had passed and I had already experienced wonderful opportunities; however, I was drained from the long hours and physical demands of nursing. I was drained from the political nuances of working in large healthcare organizations. I was drained from being surrounded by a growing number of new grads who seemed more interested in the title than learning the ropes to become strong clinical nurses. I needed a change. I was no longer serving people; I was serving a job that I was finding more and more difficult to show up to day in and day out.

Mental, emotional, and physical fatigue began to set in; yet, I felt stuck. Nursing was all I knew as far as a career goes. I contemplated changing professions; however, I wasn't interested in learning anything new (outside of the nursing profession). My growing frustration took its toll, and my ministry was turning into misery. When you operate from a place of passionless duty, the work becomes less about those you're serving and more of a chore by which we simply go through the motions for the sake of getting it done. It was time for a change.

With our expertise, there are many, many career paths nurses can take to fulfill our purpose. Yet, we often pigeonhole ourselves into only pursuing nursing opportunities that fit into the fixed perception of what a nurse does. This is part of the reason I continued to work part-time at the bedside after deciding to transition to nursing education full time. This was due in part to the necessity of supplemental income (nursing education tends to pay significantly less than bedside nursing); but mostly I felt the need to remain at the bedside to maintain my status as a 'real nurse'. I didn't want to lose my prestige and most importantly the title of RN. It's funny the limitations we place on ourselves for no good reason at all.

I finally started to realize that what I did with my profession was not nearly as important as how I did it. Nursing and healthcare can be very disparaging when you realize profit margins are considered much more than patient safety. Money drives delivery of healthcare as well as healthcare education. My disdain for the 'profit-over-people' mentality is what led me to look beyond my needs and my wants to advance the nursing profession. My priorities shifted from simply wanting to get as much as I could from this career to wanting to contribute as much as I could to uplift my own community.

Fulfilling my purpose became my number one priority. I wanted to create financial freedom so I could eventually pursue other passions I have for helping and uplifting others. I decided entrepreneurship was the best and most efficient way to create an income stream that would allow for financial and time freedom; so, I started my journey in an unconventional fashion. I didn't know anything about entrepreneurship, so I looked for what I thought would be "easy" entry points into self-employment. My first attempt at entrepreneurship was through multilevel marketing (MLM). I've sold beauty products, health supplements, legal services, and financial planning products. I thought MLM would be the vehicle to everything I wanted – freedom and passive income. The idea was good, and was doable; however, I was leading with the wrong perspective – money. My focus was to earn cash as quickly as possible with minimal investment of time and financial resources. Though I thought I was being selfless because my "why" was to create a lifestyle that would allow me to give back to others, the motive was all about me. I didn't choose any of these business types to help and serve others; I started them to increase my profits and income for self. Leading with money is not the way to start a business.

Four businesses later, I was even more disconnected from my purpose and no better off financially than before. Discouragement and lack of confidence began to take a toll on my health and lifestyle. Even amid me trying to figure things out in my entrepreneurial journey, I continued to climb the ladder in my professional role and eventually snagged an Administrator position for a local nursing education program. By all accounts, I was "successful". My career boasted a six-figure salary with a title and job responsibility I had worked hard to attain. Those around me thought I had it made – career, family, home. I was living the American dream; yet, I was still unfulfilled because what I really wanted was not in reach.

Yes, I had a husband, but we barely saw each other because I worked so much. Yes, I had beautiful children and a place to call home; but I was gone so much that even when I was home, I couldn't be present as I was too busy answering work calls and emails. Yes, I was making great money, but who had time to enjoy it? I can count on one hand the number of family trips or vacations I enjoyed with my loved ones before starting my first profitable business. I was too busy creating a life that I couldn't really live. I reached back to an important life lesson I had learned early in my career and had somehow lost sight of – money cannot buy happiness and should never be the sole reason for staying in a position of lackluster living.

While my corporate position was challenging and unfulfilling, it was a blessing in that I found my true calling in the work I was performing. Sometimes, we find our calling amid our challenges. I loved the work I was doing and was proud of the accomplishments I had achieved. I realized how good I was in my industry. I used the time in my corporate job to hone my skills for my next move. I decided to not only leave my job, but to leave the 'E' quadrant. Those of you who are fans of Robert Kiyosaki know what I mean by 'E' quadrant (if you haven't read *Cashflow Quadrant* by Kiyosaki, I suggest you do so). I wanted out of the 'employee' zone. I was confident that my next move from employment would be entrepreneurship. With an ignited passion and determination to create the life I wanted, I began the journey that eventually led me to permanently fire my boss.

My decision to venture, again, into entrepreneurship was unwavering. I was determined to build a business around my passion. An enormous weight was lifted from my shoulders, and that's when I learned the importance of simply making a decision – a decision to show up for myself. I shifted my mindset from "employee" to "employME". I began to work on my transition to business owner while still working my 9-to-5 gig. I continued to perform my work duties as required; however, I made a serious shift in priorities outside normal business hours. Instead of using my evenings and weekends to answer emails and put out fires for my boss, I used that time to work on my business. Lunch breaks were used to meet with potential clients. In fact, the road to securing my first contractual corporate client began over lunch with a key decision maker within the company. I set weekly and monthly goals and remained steadfast in reaching those goals. I convinced myself through positive self-talk and affirmations that I was already the boss and CEO to my own company – even before creating my business entity or landing my first paying client.

My entire walk changed. When I say walk, I mean my entire demeanor. I refused to stress over the workload in my job and began to walk in faith that I would manifest every business goal. To-do items for my business began to replace extracurricular work activities on my calendar. My business partner and I met weekly to review and renew our plan of action. We created victory after victory with consistency. Week after week there were new breakthroughs in our business; and I don't mean huge victories. I mean the little things such as logo creation, development of the company mission statement, completing the company website, and setup of company email. Before long, I was ready to market my business. Within six months of deciding to open my business, I landed my first paid contract. Within three months of registering my business with the secretary of state, I quit my job and opened the doors to my career training school. Four months later, I was depositing nearly $10,000 into my business account – the first paid invoice from a corporate partner (I still have a picture of the check).

The know-how of starting and running a business was not the biggest challenge of creating a six-figure business; the greatest challenge was staying the course to show up for myself every single day. I believe anyone can learn to start and grow a successful business. The major difference between those who do and those who don't is not the 'F' word (failure), it's the 'C' word (consistency). I came to realize no one would show up for me until I did – no customer, business partner, or contractual client. I had to develop and maintain the confidence that I could do it; I could build a profitable business if I only remained consistent. So many times, would-be entrepreneurs miss the mark simply because they stop doing the things to realize the goal. Successful businesses don't happen by chance – you must make it happen. The behind-the-scenes work is where all the magic happens; the stuff that no one talks about in business are the most important components to starting your business. Business ownership and growth are byproducts of consistent effort.

You see, one decision changed the trajectory of my life forever. That decision fueled the action needed to realize a profitable business. It was the decision to not only own my own business, but to conquer a goal I had dreamt of for so long. Most importantly, I wanted to help people. More than ever I wanted to help others, and I found a business that would allow me to do so using gifts and talents I already possessed. Yes, I had failed before. I was afraid of failing again; however, I was more afraid of living in regret. As a nurse, I had witnessed many people on their death beds with thoughts of wouldas, couldas, and shouldas. I didn't want my life to end with all my gifts and passions locked away in a silo of fears; and I certainly didn't want to risk wasting a gift that has the potential to help others realize their gifts. The most ultimate form of selfishness is locking away the tools you possess to help someone else overcome their challenges. I truly believe we overcome the hell of our own situations to help others do the same.

More nurses are realizing the impact of their skills, talents, and knowledge and are deciding to use those skills to open businesses. Nursing entrepreneurship empowers and advances the profession while impacting our communities locally and nationally. Alternative models of care, advanced technology, innovative ideas for healthcare education, and increased patient diversity are factors driving nurses to serve beyond the bedside through entrepreneurship. It's time we take inventory of our skills and knowledge and create businesses which impact our communities.

Nurses are in a unique position to start successful businesses using our skills.[iii] Consider this: if we, as minority women, can beat the odds and join the ranks of a profession which has less than 10% representation of those who look like us, certainly we can learn the ins and outs of starting and running a business. The history of African-American people, specifically of African-American women, is one of perseverance despite the most horrific of obstacles and circumstances. We have always found a way to turn what was given to us into something greater. Now more than ever, we need to tap into that tremendous energy and power to lay a foundation of wealth creation and community building through entrepreneurship.

So, why leave your nice pay, benefits, and prestige of nursing to open your own business? Perhaps you want to elevate your earning potential and create more autonomy around your earnings. Did you know black nurses tend to earn less wages than their white counterparts? The mean hourly wage for black nurses in the U.S. is $31.92 compared to a mean wage of $33.02 for white nurses.[iv] Maybe you'd like to have more time, freedom, and control over your schedule. Sometimes, I think we like the idea of having the title of boss, entrepreneur, or business owner more than we understand what it really means to be an entrepreneur.

Entrepreneurship is about service. I started my business out of a desire to provide a service to minority youth that wasn't provided to me while growing up. When we look for ways to serve those around us, profit and increase will follow. As a nursing entrepreneur, you find yourself in a unique position to serve from a place that only a nurse can. Decide the service you want to provide, and the rest will follow. When you serve, you create an overflow of abundance for your business, yourself, and those you serve.

So, what does it take to make it to the top of your game in business and beyond? I'm often asked these questions: "How did you start your business?" and "What inspired you to start your business?" The truth of the matter is business start-up is a lot like nursing school. You go into it not knowing what to expect. It is unchartered territory for you, yet you find a way to navigate through uncertainty and self-doubt. You create support systems and surround yourself with others on the same journey and a few who have been on the journey and have achieved some level of success. We can do anything we put our minds to; this is the beauty of the human experience. *Starting* my business was not a challenge; the real challenge was *deciding* that I would step out on faith and ...well – start. In this information age, the 'how-to' is not really the issue. You can do a quick internet search and have a business entity setup and ready to market within 24 hours or less. Literally.

So, if the 'how-to' is not the right question to ask about taking the leap of faith toward entrepreneurship, then what question should we be asking? What's the secret sauce that led a teen mom from public housing and public assistance to not only finish college, but to eventually earn a Master's degree in her field? A young woman who was victim to physical, sexual, and emotional abuse for a significant portion of her childhood now runs a six-figure business. She, a product of a single parent home, now enjoys a life she could only dream of and hope for.

Against all odds, she's defined success for herself – by herself. This is the epitome of making power moves while no one is looking.

The truth is there is no secret sauce. The universe has an abundance of resources for each of us to tap into, if we so choose. It is as simple as positioning yourself to prosper on every level through your determination that it will be done. Do not allow others to place their limitations on your life. I almost allowed others' limited views of what a nurse is "supposed" to look like hinder me from using my skills to charter a different path in my career. Taking the road least traveled sounds like a noble concept; however, it does not come without resistance. You must take responsibility for your own happiness and allow yourself to remain in passionate pursuit of that happiness no matter what. You will not have all the answers; move forward anyway. You'll feel lonely and out of sorts at times; keep pushing anyway. Someone will tell you to just quit and do something easier; pursue your dream anyway. Someone else's impossible isn't your problem; don't own that type of limitation in your life. The world's greatest inventions came from people who didn't let impossibilities stop them. We never thought it possible to be airborne or to study life on other planets – until someone else did it first.

What I have learned on this journey is that, sometimes, the ones who make it to the top are the very people others never saw coming. I was invisible to many – until I wasn't. Nice girls don't always finish last; and the least among us are often the most powerful. Nursing entrepreneurship is more than a proclamation of "boss status", "Nurse CEO", or "business babe". The hashtags and social media frenzy surrounding entrepreneurship these days is overwhelming. Unrealistic images are tainting the view of entrepreneurship. Some of us are getting a perception about the view from a birds-eye perspective. Allow me to introduce the two most important concepts that have led to success in business and life: serve and show up.

The capacity in which we serve must match our hustle and the focus we put on advancing ourselves. We cannot commit to service through entrepreneurship without committing to providing the type of service we'd want for ourselves. This means showing up each day with an attitude of doing work that is beyond your wants and desires. Yes, we need to make money in our business to survive; however, leading with money makes us vultures rather than trailblazers. The little girl from Gary I once knew has taken the focus away from her needs and now creates products which provide for the needs of others. It's very easy to get caught up in the selfish ambition that often drives a person to success. We can become so consumed with getting more for ourselves – more money, material possessions, or notoriety. What does it mean to profit if you lose yourself in the process? Do the work; seize every opportunity to grow; show yourself grace on this journey; and, above all, challenge yourself to show up every day – for others and for yourself.

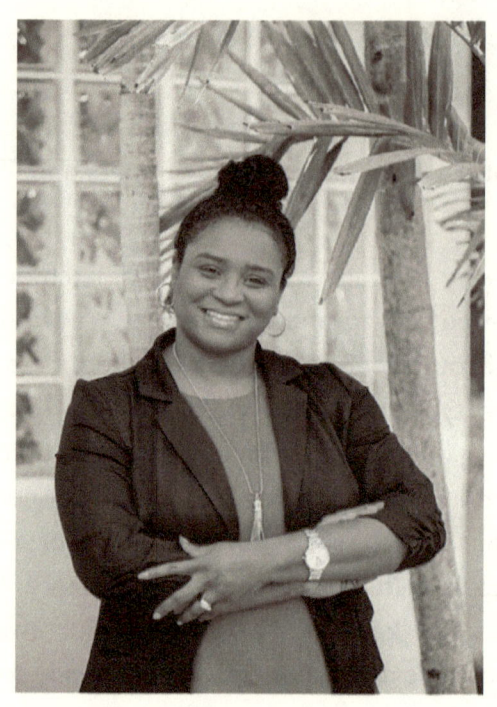

About the Author

A native of Gary, Indiana, Brandi London is a Registered Nurse of more than 15 years. She obtained her Bachelor's of Science in Nursing from Indiana University Northwest in 2002, and her Master's of Science in Nursing and Healthcare Education from the University of Phoenix in 2011. Brandi's Nursing experience covers a variety of acute care and academic settings. Her desire to provide quality healthcare education for minorities lead her to leave her corporate job to pursue entrepreneurship. Brandi is a full-time, serial entrepreneur. She is co-founder of Hardon Educational Institute, LLC, a healthcare career training company, and is a founding partner of a local home health agency. In addition, Brandi is founder of Nurse Biz Mogul, LLC where she serves as a Business Strategist, helping nurses and other healthcare professionals transition from employee to entrepreneur. She is an active member of Sigma Gamma Rho Sorority, Inc. Brandi is married to her husband of 16 years, Damian, and has three sons – Jalen, Jamari, and Jamir. In her spare time, Brandi enjoys spending time with family and traveling.

To Contact The Author:

Email: admin@Nursebizmogul.com

FB: Nurse Biz Mogul

Instagram: @Nursebizmogul

Twitter: @Nursebizmogul

BEYOND THE BEDSIDE

Dr. Jesslyn Anderson, FNP-C

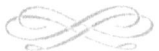

INTRODUCTION:

I remember, as a little girl, seeing my mom put on a crisp white uniform, white stockings, and white shoes before kissing me and heading out to work. I thought she was a nurse until I found out when I was older that she worked as an EKG technician in the ER. It didn't matter she oozed passion for what she did; and, looking back, I know that is why I chose the career path I did. My mind was made up and I never wavered from the seed that was planted in me early on to become a Registered Nurse. When I graduated from high school, I was accepted into Presbyterian School of Nursing and my journey to becoming a nurse was underway.

The summer before starting nursing school, one of my cousins convinced me to work with her for the summer at a factory. She helped me to get hired on and I was excited to be making $6.50/hr. The job was repetitive and not very challenging at all, but the people were nice, and I was getting a check. It was taxing on the body because we stood for eight hours a day packing individual batteries in boxes. There were times I felt like herded cattle, the breaks were timed down to the second, and I did not enjoy the work. Looking back, I have always been grateful for that experience because it gave me a greater appreciation and respect for earning my degree. I admired the individuals that worked there but for me I understood very well what I needed to do and what I had no desire to ever do again.

I started Presbyterian School of Nursing in the fall of 1996. My first semester of nursing school was by far the hardest and the first time in my life I had to truly study to get good grades. The graciousness of making up tests to replace a low grade, which I was used to from my high school teachers, was replaced with indifference from my college professors. I will never forget making a 67 on my first anatomy test. I was literally in shock! My professor gave back my failed test with the grade and corresponding alphabet written in red ink on it like the boss of the classroom she was. The majority of the class failed and she made it clear the grade would not be replaced. She let it be known that if we wanted to pass her class, we needed to buckle down.

I was a little shell-shocked by that experience, but being a poor black girl from the "wrong side of the tracks", failing was not an option for me. My future was riding on this and I could not let my family down. I thought about my grandmother and a conversation we had once. I saw my grandmother crying on the couch one day, her tears soaking her face. I hated to see my grandmother cry but that day it was tears of pride. She talked about having to drop out of school in the eighth grade. She grew up in the Jim Crow South where the dreams of little black boys and girls were snuffed out with the scourge of racism. She married young and never had the opportunity to return to school. She had worked various jobs to take care of her children and put food on the table and knew that she wanted better for her children and grandchildren. I was the first one in my family to go to college and she knew her sacrifices made it possible. She told me how proud she was of me for starting college in the fall and needed me to make her one promise. She needed me to promise that I would graduate so I would not have to work as hard as she did. My grandmother and dad would repeatedly say, "Once you get your education, they cannot take that away from you". My grandmother may not have been rich in the sense of worldly goods, but she was rich in love, care, support, and wisdom that money could never buy. Above all, she was a prayer warrior and looking back over my life I know her prayers sustained and propelled me.

Early on in life, I developed a drive to succeed even when the odds were stacked against me. I was one of four African Americans in a class of fifty plus students when I started nursing school. Anyone that has ever been to nursing school knows the first two semesters are used to weed out students. I was a survivor...had been all my life. Even under insurmountable odds, I always kept the faith and understood the promise. I was determined to finish nursing school and three looooooonnnnnngggg hard years later, I'm telling you the STRUGGLE WAS REAL, I graduated with my Diploma in Nursing. I was the first one to graduate from college, so it was a CELEBRATION!!!! My entire family was there to watch me walk across the stage and it was an important moment in our family's history. Graduating gave me a sense of accomplishment I had never felt before. I took my NCLEX and recall how nerve-wracking it was waiting for my results. I was on vacation celebrating my graduation when my results came in the mail. My mom and grandmother called to tell me my results had come in the mail. The anticipation was too much and I needed to know. The results were in and I PASSED! Finally, I had fulfilled my childhood dream of becoming a nurse. Like I was really a nurse, like a REAL NURSE... an actual REGISTERED

NURSE.

I decided to complete an additional year of school to obtain my BSN. While I was completing my degree, I became pregnant with my son. This was disappointing to my parents and grandmother, but I made the best of the situation. My Sonshine was born a few weeks before I finished my last semester of school. I was out for one week and returned the next week, much to the surprise of my classmates and teachers, but I could not afford to withdraw or miss my final exams. In August 2000, I completed my BSN. I was given an option to continue for one additional year and obtain my MSN but I had a little baby that required my undivided attention.

Two years passed before I even thought about going back to school again. I applied for the Family Nurse Practitioner program at a local university. I was not accepted into the program but given the option to begin taking courses toward the program as a post-baccalaureate student. That was the first time I had applied for something academically and was denied. A part of me felt like a failure, but little did I know my degree was DELAYED not DENIED. At that time, we only had a handful of nurse practitioners (NPs) where I worked and the pay was paltry. Besides by this time, I had met my future husband and was head over heels. We were traveling and enjoying life so needless to say I had gotten a little sidetracked.

In the fall of 2006, I enrolled in a Master of Business Administration (MBA) program. This was my first time being introduced to the business side of healthcare. The information I learned in my MBA program was invaluable. I learned about contract law, how to write a business plan, developing strategic partnerships, and marketing to prospective clients. I had the knowledge, but I was still missing the detailed know how and practical real-world application. I graduated in 2008 when the recession was underway. This was the first time the healthcare industry was affected since I started my career and overtime was not as plentiful. Foolishly - because I did not understand investing - I went into conservation mode financially. Looking back I realized I missed out on a prime opportunity to invest in real estate.

Boredom and upheaval on my job led to me try travel nursing for about a year. While I liked the money, I did not like being on the road and away from my family. I begin to think about the next phase of my nursing career. After 12 years, I had grown weary of bedside nursing. I daydreamed about being an entrepreneur but I was not uncomfortable enough to make a change. I applied to become a nurse on my company's resource team. As a member of the resource team, I could take "mini assignments" throughout the organization on units that needed help for a few weeks to a few months and the hourly pay was comparable to the pay I was making traveling. It was a win-win situation for me because my pocketbook felt like I was a travel nurse without some of the drawbacks of being a travel nurse. It increased my knowledge, expanded my nursing skills, and opened me up to areas of nursing I had never worked in before. I continued to daydream about opening my own business and seriously ponder going back to school to become a NP. I signed up for my local college's business center seminars and started considering nurse practitioner schools.

I attended several small business workshops but was still paralyzed by fear. I also did not have a solid idea of what kind of business I wanted to pursue. I would daydream about being successful in business, but the thought of stepping into the unknown was scary. I wanted to feel safe, so I fell back to what I knew and was comfortable with - going to school. I knew how to do that well. I had gone to school so much by then my family and friends begin to tease me about being a career student. School was a familiar comfort zone in which I knew I could succeed and win. In my mind, it was a guaranteed win. I knew I would receive the course outline, syllabus, expectations, and assignments. The rhythm of school was so familiar to me and was safer than stepping out and starting a business. I decided becoming a NP would be my next career move.

I finally settled on the University of Cincinnati after a recommendation from a friend and started in 2013. Since I had a previous master's degree, I was able to get credit for two courses. I doubled up on my classes the first semester so I could eliminate an entire semester and finish early. Nurse Practitioner school was challenging, and I welcomed the challenge. It was definitely a learning curve and for the first time in a long time, I felt like a newbie. I was out of my comfort zone and my nerves were frazzled when it finally hit me the amount of responsibility that would come with this new role. I graduated with honors the following year and passed boards the following month. Also during this time, there was lots of discussion on Facebook about the Doctorate of Nursing Practice (DNP) degree. I begin to consider doing this and knew if I stayed out of school too long I was done. I started looking for a job, applied for a spot in my organization's fellowship program, and applied to Chatham's DNP program.

I was hustling at this point and had a plan A, B, and C and a backup plan to those. I received the job offer, was accepted into the DNP program, and a few months later was accepted into the fellowship program. All I could think was LOOK AT GOD! I could not do all of them so I put the DNP program on hold and started my first job as a nurse practitioner.

I really liked my first job as a NP but I needed to decide on the fellowship program. The fellowship program was a one-year advance care provider (ACP) program that operated much like a medical residency program, but it came with a significant pay cut.

I discussed it with my hubby and prayed about it. He gave me the assurance that he would be supportive of any decision I made but most of the financial burden would be on him again if I went into the fellowship. My job had its pros but the fellowship program would be invaluable to my career. DECISIONS, DECISIONS, DECISIONS! I did not make a decision until I felt an overwhelming peace with one of the choices. With an answer from God, I knew it was the best decision for my career.

I had delayed starting the DNP program until later that year. Family and friends thought I was crazy to enroll in a DNP program full-time and continue with the fellowship program full-time. I was in BEAST MODE! It was tough and there were times I wanted to quit but I kept my eye on the prize. I finished the fellowship program and a few months later my Doctorate of Nursing Practice (DNP). It felt surreal. Was I dreaming? Dr. Jesslyn Anderson definitely had a nice ring to it! When I received my degree in the mail, I visited my grandmother's grave so I could dedicate it to her. She made the ultimate sacrifice in more ways than one and I would not be where I am today if not for her.

After I completed my DNP degree, I took a mental break. I decided to rest and do nothing. The previous four years were grueling and I needed some time to do absolutely nothing. I savored that time off. I spent time with my family, worked, traveled, and led a "normal" life with no deadlines, syllabus, papers or assignments due. I begin to think a lot about starting a business and knew my future would involve entrepreneurship. I eventually settled on the idea of opening a mobile house calls practice.

I had a little bit of business knowledge from the business seminars I had attended and information I had been gathering over the years. My main issue was FEAR. I had to deal with the fear that had me paralyzed. Fear of starting a business, fear of failure, fear of the unknown, just life draining FEAR - and I was operating in it. Fear had its death grips on me for many reasons, and it was holding me back from being intentional and purposeful. I wanted to become an entrepreneur to secure freedom in my life and finances. I desire to be at a point in life where I work, not because I have to, but because I want to. I will never have the freedom I covet working for someone else.

In early 2017, I started to pray about and truly deal with the fear that was keeping me stuck. I was able to connect with and join various business groups on Facebook. I took time to read, research, and ask questions from more seasoned business owners. I joined a business group and started taking more meaningful steps towards opening a business. The first "business" I started was a t-shirt printing business. I had no intention of starting this side hustle and originally purchased the equipment for my son. I was excited for him and willing to support his dream only to realize he wasn't as interested in making t-shirts as he pretended to be when he asked me to invest my money. I purchased all the equipment he needed only for it to sit untouched for almost two months. Little did I know that supporting my son would lead me down the path to my own entrepreneurial endeavor.

One day I decided to take the equipment out and learn how to make shirts myself. My first t-shirt design came out better than I expected, so I started making them for my family for free initially. Shortly after that at the urging of a cousin, I designed our family reunion t-shirts. I was going to send the design to the business we had picked to print our shirts but my cousin encouraged me to make them instead. I was nervous because it was such a large order and scared my family would be critical of them. The shirts were a hit. My family loved them and this helped to build my confidence. I decided not to advertise from fear of becoming overwhelmed with orders and getting sidetracked from starting my dream business. I have never advertised this on social media and any business I get is strictly word of mouth. I continue to print custom t-shirts with the help of my husband and have thought about expanding into e-commerce. While I am thankful God opened this door, I still had another business goal in mind.

I remained laser-focused on my main goal of opening a mobile house calls practice. The model is sustaining and a profitable niche in the healthcare industry. People are looking for convenience and affordable healthcare options. I reached out to friends that owned their own businesses for advice. I followed various nurse entrepreneur groups on Facebook more closely. It was inspiring to see so many African American women that were running successful businesses. That old adage "seeing is believing" is true. I would search the group for valuable resources, answers to some of my business questions, and upcoming webinars. The ease of connecting with individuals who want to do, are doing, or have already accomplished what you are seeking to do was a game changer for me. When I looked back over my career, I realized I had been preparing myself for this moment for years. Everything I had done up to this point from obtaining my MBA degree, attending business seminars, and making strategic connections prepared me for this moment.

In late 2017, I started taking concrete steps to open my own house calls practice. A strategic connection I had with a fellow NP was how I found my supervising MD. I can recall the first meeting I had with him about developing a partnership. I was so nervous and feared his answer would be no. On the contrary, our first meeting went well, and he said YES! That was a huge moment in my journey. I can recall being overwhelmed and shedding tears of joy. I was excited but it was scary too. The next month I allowed fear to creep back in. Instead of moving forward diligently, I started taking my time on purpose. The idea of being a business owner and being responsible for EVERYTHING was starting to scare me. I started to second guess myself and ask if this was what I really wanted. I called up a friend whom I respect, admire, and have known for a long time for advice. She had to remind me that entrepreneurship is scary; but if your dreams do not scare you, then they are not big enough. I needed that pep talk to get back in line with my vision and continue to pursue my dream. I begin to meet with my supervising MD monthly so he could track my progress, answer any questions, and provide me with resources if needed. OnSite Care will officially be open for business this year. I am in my final trimester and getting ready to PUSH!!!!

I am just beginning my journey into entrepreneurship. At this point in my story, I have experienced more triumphs than trials. The biggest obstacles I had to overcome were fear and second-guessing myself. I operated in fear too long and needed to start walking by faith. Fear can be paralyzing. It will keep you stuck in the daydreaming phase of your vision. I'm not saying you will be completely fearless. Stepping into the unknown and being unsure of yourself is absolutely scary. I still get twinges of fear from time to time, but it does not stop me from moving forward any longer. Rational fear is a normal part of the process. I am learning to trust my instincts more and be ok with missteps. I have accepted that I am new at this and just like a baby that begins to walk I will stumble and fall a few times as I continue to learn.

Here are a few pearls that have helped me along the way:

1. FAITH over fear always. Trust God and trust the process.

2. Don't be afraid to ASK God for what you want and SPEAK your vision(s) into the universe.

3. Write down your goals and review them periodically.

4. Locate your local small business administration center and sign up to get alerts for seminars and workshops.

5. Research, research, and research some more.

6. When you think you have found an answer to your question, go back and research it again. Your business and wallet will thank you!

7. Don't be afraid to ask questions and seek advice from others.

8. Join local and social media business groups and NETWORK, NETWORK, NETWORK.

9. Expensive does not always mean better. Watch them coins!

10. THINK BIG. Your business goals should scare you!

As I have been on this journey called life, one thing I truly understand is that everything has a purpose, place, time, and season. There is an old African proverb that says, "When you pray, move your feet". I have prayed and now I'm moving. I am excited and nervous about what God has in store for me in the coming months and years. This has been an amazing year of learning and growth for me. I am thankful for every opportunity, any disappointments, and even for the missteps and mishaps that have come my way. I am grateful for my husband, family, and close friends who have been nothing but supportive of me on this journey. This year, I am declaring new heights will be reached in my business; I will be blessed beyond measure; everything I touch will turn to gold; I will develop strategic partnerships that will bless me abundantly; my cup will overflow, I will remain humble, have a spirit of giving, and; never forget where I started. Reaching back is a must. I would not be where I am today if not for the sacrifices of those that came before me. I AM MY ANCESTOR'S WILDEST DREAMS!!!!!

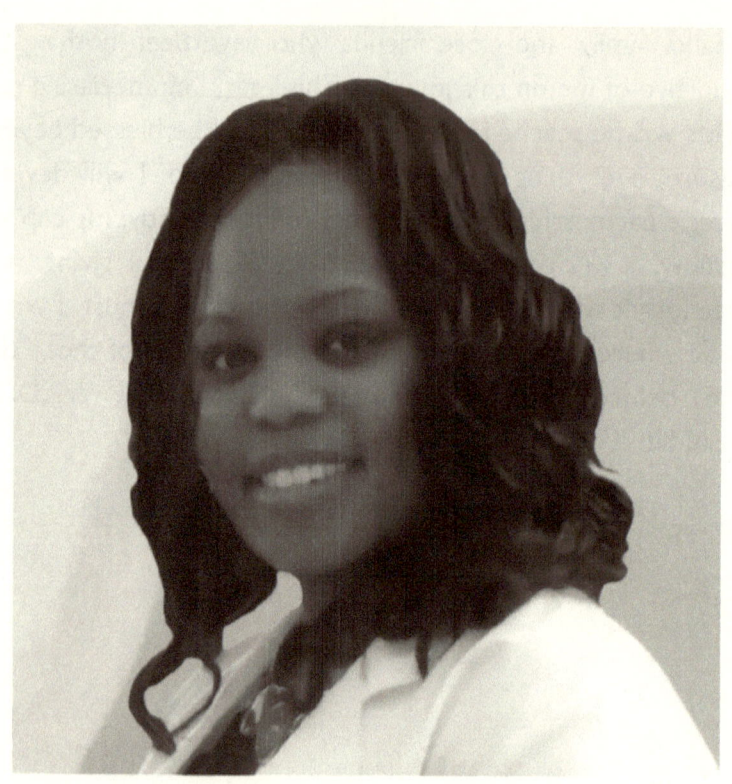

About the Author

Jesslyn Anderson, DNP, MBA/HCM, FNP-C is a native of Rock Hill, SC and resides there with her husband and son. She has enjoyed a long career in healthcare working as a RN for over 15 years before becoming a Nurse Practitioner in 2014. She received her Bachelor of Science in Nursing from Queen's University, her MBA with a specialization in healthcare management from University of Phoenix, her Master of Science in Nursing from University of Cincinnati, and her Doctorate of

Nursing from Chatham University. She currently works full-time as a Nurse Practitioner at a local hospital in Charlotte, NC. She is pursuing her dream of becoming a CEO and currently working towards opening On-Site Care, a mobile house calls practice, in 2018.She has a passion for patient education, improving health outcomes and addressing health disparities in minority populations. In her free time, she enjoys traveling and spending time with her family.

To Contact The Author

EMAIL: info@onsitecarellc.com

LIPSTICK AND STETHOSCOPES

Portia "Revlon" Wofford

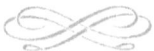

At the beginning of 2017, I had an epiphany and wrote a mantra on my Facebook page: "I have the Midas touch, this year. Everything and everyone that I encounter will flourish!" I wrote this mantra with the goal to inspire others, but I really needed to inspire myself. I was so tired of going through the motions of life. I had a purpose that needed to be fulfilled. I'd survived so much that life had thrown at me; I knew that I needed more fulfillment in my career. I was empty and tired of being a glorified pill pusher. I lacked enthusiasm for my career and had started considering other career options. Nursing was where my heart was; however, what else could I do to touch lives and still feel complete? Entrepreneurship had been on my to-do list since the day I passed the NCLEX. I knew working for someone else was not what I wanted to do. I wanted a legacy for my son and generations to come. I knew entrepreneurship would be the only way to obtain my goal.

I'm Portia; however, you may know me as Revlon. Revlon is a name that was bestowed upon me by a former coworker. I was the typical new nurse; excited to have my first "big girl job"; excited at the opportunity to make more than the minimum wage I was making at Walmart. More than anything, however, I had the chance to change lives. I would come into work with my crisp scrubs and makeup slayed. I never missed a beat. One of my coworkers told me, "You look like a Revlon model. I'm going to call you Revlon!" Well, as all things do in small towns, the name spread. Before long residents and their families were calling me "Revlon". It stuck, and it became a sobriquet. I loved it and saw it as an alter ego. Revlon was pretty, sophisticated, and intelligent. She was confident. She was everything I pretended to be.

The adage is true that the son will pay for the father's sins. Well, in my case the daughter paid for the mother's sins. My mother gave birth to me at the young age of sixteen. I was the eldest of three children that she bore before she turned 21. I don't think she was ever really ready to be a mother. She was young and naive- so young and naive, she often chose another life over her children. This eventually led to my brother, sister, and I being taken from her. I will never forget the moment we were escorted away from our home, in the projects, by a social worker and a police officer to a foster home. Life inside the foster home was hell for me. I was tormented and physically abused by the older girls. If I didn't eat quickly enough I was pinched. If I ate too quickly I was kneed, under the table. I began to wet the bed, and this only escalated the abuse. I realized that people will disappoint you and that it was up to me to change the course of my life. I had learned that reporting the abuse, to the mother of the house, would do me no good. Instead of being protected, I was scolded and warned not to be a tattletale. I recall one night being awakened by cold, ice water thrown on me. Instead of tattling, I got out of bed, changed the sheets and my clothes, got back into bed, and silently cried myself to sleep. I was four or five and I had already learned to be self-reliant and self-preserving. I learned to take care of myself and to just get things done. It was in that foster home, that I learned to be independent. Later, in life, these characteristics would serve me well, despite their terrible origins.

After leaving the foster home, my two siblings and I were raised by a single father, with the help of our grandparents. My dad hung the moon! He was the type of father who braided hair, taught us how to throw a softball, and provided for us in the best way he could. My mother did not have a major role, if any, in my life. All the things that a mother is supposed to teach a daughter I learned on my own or from one of the many surrogate mothers I had. My trust of women was nonexistent. All too often, I was reminded of it and the feelings of hate and disgust that some of my family members had towards my mother were deflected onto me. By the age of ten, I was experiencing suicidal ideations. I was depressed and experiencing anxiety. I excelled academically as this was the only way that I received any form of praise and relief from the mental and emotional abuse that I endured almost daily. I was determined to make something out of myself. I did not want to be known as my mother's daughter. I was constantly reminded I would not amount to anything and I was worthless. I knew getting an education and working hard to excel at a career was my only way out. I graduated at the top of my class and everyone had the highest expectations for me. I was set on the path to gain multiple degrees, land a government job, and live the fabulous life. Then, LIFE HAPPENED, and I was sent on a slow spiraling path of disappointment, failure, and depression. All through high school, I had aspired to become a forensic scientist. Nursing was not on my radar at all. I majored in criminal justice and English. I was so severely depressed - as I had been most of my life - and was struggling to overcome feelings of inadequacy, doubt, and guilt. I carried those feeling with me off to college. In November, of my freshman year, my great-grandmother died. Her death impacted me negatively. She was the glue which held our family together and she and I were very close. The semester was coming to an end and I had no idea how I was going to pay for my next semester. My dad couldn't afford my tuition and my Pell Grant wasn't enough to cover it. I had emptied my savings account as I had to help pay for my first semester's tuition. I was worried constantly and the stress of school left me ill most days. I went home for the Christmas and New Year holidays and the heaviness of the pain my Big Mama's death had caused coupled with the stress of not being able to pay for the next semester and a bad breakup of my first "adult" relationship weighed heavily on my mind and heart; I decided to attempt suicide. I sat in my Granny's bathtub, took 20 extra strength Tylenol and chased them with a shot of cranberry juice and Vodka. I filled the bathtub up with water and prayed I would drift off to sleep and drown peacefully. As I was lying, in that tub my life flashed before my eyes. All the disappointment, fear, anxiety, and anguish that I had experienced was one breath away from being gone. I was one breath away from never feeling the hurt and pain again.

A family friend rushed me to the local emergency room and I was eventually rushed to a bigger hospital. I spent two weeks in the hospital. Five of those days were in the ICU. I became obsessed with the nurses. I envied their compassion for others, studied their movements and habits, and was intrigued by their enthusiasm for their job and my life. These people whom I did not know and whom had never previously spoken two words to me were showing me so much compassion and empathy. Every day on every shift, my nurses encouraged me to get better. They listened to me and encouraged me to live. When I was finally discharged home, I had no idea if I wanted to live; but I would remember the words of the nurses and I knew that nursing was the career for me.

Fast forward to the age of 20. I had taken some time off from the university I attended, but I knew college was my ultimate goal. By this time, I was in a relationship with an older man and he encouraged me to go after my dreams. I enrolled in the local community college; however, I found myself pregnant while in college. Something that I always said I wouldn't be. Here I was again, disappointing myself and everyone around me. I was ashamed. I was another statistic. A single, black woman with no education, working at Walmart. How was I going to take care of a baby? My pregnancy was horrible. I experienced hyperemesis gravida and had to be hospitalized for dehydration several times. I struggled to get through my classes, but nevertheless I progressed. I would go to class, leave for my doctor's appointments, and then go back to class. It was difficult and trying, but I knew I had to accomplish my goal. I refused to be a statistic. At this time, I was pursuing a Criminal Justice and English degree. After giving birth prematurely, I realized that pursuing those degrees was no longer rational and I needed a career that was convenient, steady, and could afford me the lifestyle I always wanted. I prematurely gave birth to a baby boy at twenty-eight weeks on a Thursday and returned to class on Monday. My baby was still in the hospital, so I would go to class, leave, and return to the hospital. I knew I could not continue school, work, and motherhood simultaneously for another two or three years. I had to find another route to accomplish my goal of having a career.

I often tell the story of how volunteering in a nursing home and shadowing the nurses is what persuaded me to become a nurse; however, finding myself pregnant while in college and giving birth prematurely left me desperate. I would often think back to how the nurses in the ICU treated me. I knew what I had to do. I applied for the Practical Nursing program and I was accepted. I still was not sure this was the career path for me, but I was excited to be accepted. My family was not as excited. They questioned why I didn't apply for the Registered Nursing program instead. Even now, I often think back to that time of my life and wonder why I didn't pursue that route. My thought process back then was to get through school, quickly, so I could make more money and spend more time with my son. I don't regret it. Nursing school was the most difficult thing I have ever endured. I often joke and say it was more difficult than childbirth. I recall sitting in my bed one night, books in one hand and my son in the other. I had a vision. The vision was of me walking into the room of a girl who had attempted suicide. I spoke with her and encouraged her. I knew then that nursing was for me. I was being given a platform - a platform where I would have access to those who truly needed me. I could save lives. I could heal. I could make a difference. I knew that they day would come, that I'd have to share my story to some young girl, under my care, to save her life! I finished nursing school and landed my first job at a local nursing home.

I loved my job! I became attached to my residents and I enjoyed going to work. Three months into my new position, I became anxious. I knew I wanted more than to pass pills and chart. I knew I had to get back to school and pursue a higher nursing degree. I began taking prerequisites and was determined to enroll in an LPN to RN bridge program. I applied to a program at the local community college only to not be accepted. I was devastated. I had become bored with the monotonous tasks at work. I felt underappreciated and overwhelmed. I was working sixteen-hour shifts against my wishes; and with the new management at the facility, there was a shift to have more Registered Nurses per shift. I knew if I wanted to advance in my career or gain respect, then I needed to obtain the next degree. I needed to take and pass Anatomy & Physiology II and Microbiology to apply to a Bachelor of Science in Nursing program. At this time, I was going through a breakup and my depression and anxiety levels were up. I had panic attacks daily and could barely make it out of bed. I was depressed and experiencing suicidal ideations. I had only been a nurse for a year; however, the stress of working sixteen-hour shifts and going to school made me regret my decision. I no longer had the motivation or aspiration to continue with my education or career. I failed my anatomy class and I gave up; however, no one knew how I was feeling. I held up the facade that I was always happy.

I began experiencing bullying from my boss. She started to schedule me for sixteen-hour shifts without asking me and I was burnt out. I was still a new nurse and didn't feel as if I had earned the right to speak up for myself. Sometimes I would work 40 hours in three days. I was exhausted and mentally I did not know how much I could tolerate. I often felt disrespected at work and felt as though I was being bullied by upper management. Eventually, I began looking for another job and I landed another position. I quit my first job and began to work for another long-term care facility. I worked at this facility for a year before beginning to feel that the workplace was unsafe. The resident to nurse ratio was sometimes 40:1

and I was on a unit with dementia patients who were wanderers and would often try to elope. I felt that my nursing license was on the line every time that I clocked in. I was scared for my license, the safety of my patients, and my peace of mind. Eventually, a former coworker called me and told me that the home health agency she worked for needed a part-time LPN. She convinced me to apply and assured me that I would love the flexibility. I applied for the part-time position and landed it. I quit my job at the nursing home and was excited to expand my skills with the home health company.

I loved my home health job! I had autonomy. My skills were appreciated by my patients and their physicians. I excelled at my job. I learned new skills and became confident in my skills. I was working closely with patients, their caregivers, and their physicians. After only working a few months, my part-time position turned into a full-time position and my boss would often praise the job I was doing. I felt respected and I enjoyed educating my patients and their caregivers. Little did I know this job was the stepping stone for me to pursue entrepreneurship. Working for a home health agency challenges you to rely on yourself and your skills. It forced me to have time management and organizational skills. I had to be self-reliant, dependable, and learn to communicate with diverse groups of people. I became accustomed to speaking with physicians and being their eyes and ears out in the field. It was an experience that changed my life! It gave me the confidence to speak to authoritative figures. I learned how to make sound decisions and stand by them. A year into my position I earned another title that would give me the skills of care coordination and care management. I enjoyed it but - as always being an LPN - it left me with little room to advance within the company. I was working a day job, so going back to school was not an option. I had built a lifestyle I could not afford to lose. My son was busy with sports, extracurricular activities, and piano lessons; I did not have time for school. I was feeling empty. I had transitioned and was working with a new RN case manager whom I felt at the time did not respect my experience or knowledge. It didn't matter how I much I knew. It didn't matter that I was the constant in my patients' lives that prevented rehospitalization. She was the RN and I was just the LPN. She always had the final say.

One day, I was sitting home, charting and I said to myself, "I can do this, independently. I am the one who is keeping these patients out of the hospital. I'm the one coordinating care, educating, and performing assessments and wound care. I can do this alone." I began to plan my exit-strategy. I continued to work and picked up a part-time job at a nursing home. I knew that I didn't want to take out loans, so I worked my part-time job for revenue for my business. I had no support besides my sister; and my anxiety and panic attacks began to return. In April of 2017, I went part-time with the home health agency to prepare myself to leave. I knew that if I wanted new doors to open, I had to close the old ones. I eventually took a job with an acute care clinic and I hated it. Yet again, I found myself doing monotonous tasks which left me empty and bored. The patient load was low, and the job would often require me to travel. Having a nine years old son at home, traveling over an hour to work was out of the question. I left that job and decided to work part-time at my home health and nursing home jobs.

I sat on my idea for about five years before stepping out on faith! However, there were a few problems. I had no money, no support, and no experience! I became disheartened. After being discouraged from continuing to pursue entrepreneurship, I decided it may be better to continue to work until I saved up enough money to venture out on my own. The thoughts of having my own business continued to weigh on my heart and mind; so, I picked up tons of extra shifts. I decided not to renew my lease on my townhouse and moved into a smaller home. I had my cable turned off. I lived the most minimal life. I had to make sacrifices.

I recalled the times I would hear other nurses gossiping about me. They would say things such as, "This is not a fashion show. She's too flashy. Does she think she is a model?" I would hear those hurtful words and use them and try to fit into a mold of what I assumed a nurse should be. After launching my brand, I realized that nurses are no longer in all white with their hair pinned up. We are so much more. We can be fashionable and professional! This gave me the idea to launch an apparel line exclusively for healthcare professionals. It is also the story behind one of my brand's most recognized slogans: *Lipstick and Stethoscope(s)*. I then took a giant and terrifying leap and chose a name: *Your Nurse Connection*!

It was not an easy task. Outside of my sister, I had no support. Instead of encouraging and supporting me, those closest to me would often say things such as, "You should go back and get your RN license before trying to start a business. No one is going to respect you because you're just an LPN. You don't have the money to start a business." They were right. I had no money. However, I could not continue to sit on my dream, "until the time was right." The time would never be right! So, I started blogging, as way to fuel my passion to educate the community, while simultaneously getting my name in front of the industry. Blogging was an efficient yet inexpensive way to start building valuable relationships, as well as my brand. Blogging became one of my biggest platforms. I was able to meet other nurse bloggers who openly gave advice and placed me in positions to meet others who held great influence in the nurse entrepreneurship world. I knew I needed support and motivation, so I navigated social media and found other nurse entrepreneurs to network with via Facebook groups. It was the best decision I could have made! I often thought back to the times when I felt alone and empty within my career. I had no professional support or encouragement. Along with my anxiety, there were days I dreaded getting out of bed to go to work. I realized that as a nurse, as well as other healthcare professions, expanding your knowledge and making yourself more marketable were the keys to autonomy and fulfillment. I wanted to form an organization, like a sorority or fraternity for healthcare professionals. I also wanted to show other LPNs there is so much more. You don't have to be belittled and disrespected. You can use your skills and experiences to shape the lives of others as well as your own.

Your Nurse Connection has a mission statement of "connecting the community healthcare professionals through education, empowerment, support, and advocacy." I am passionate about connecting the community with qualified healthcare professionals by successfully equipping those healthcare professionals with the necessary tools to adequately serve his or her community. We strive to be the go-to organization for ALL healthcare professionals and to make valuable connections; aiding healthcare professionals in advancing their careers and/or businesses. Whether a healthcare professional strives to own a business or earn certifications, to advance a stagnant career, my mission is to be that bridge and close the gap. I have been able to secure those relationships and resources. I've had the privilege to work with other nurse entrepreneurs and feature them, their courses, classes, or etcetera on my platforms. This has left me with so much fulfillment. If we are happy and fulfilled, within our careers, we can save more lives.

Since the launch of *Your Nurse Connection*, my life has completely changed. It has not always been easy. I have gone through periods of doubt and wanting to give up. Sales have been slow, and the naysayers have taken over my mind at times. I have worked hard! I have had to prove that I belong. I have had to prove that LPNs belong and that we are not to be dismissed! I began to utilize social media as a marketing and networking tool before I even knew what my brand's identity was. I hired a brand strategist and she helped me to find out who I was as a business and as a businesswoman. From that moment, my brand took off! I have met some of the most inspiring women. Had I not put myself out on a limb, I would still be stuck in yet another dead-in job. I am slowly, but steadily becoming an authoritative figure and influencer, within my industry. I have had the privilege of being featured on podcasts, radio shows, blogs, and other entrepreneurs' platforms. I have landed roles as a contributor and marketing consultant for other nursing firms. I am now a published author and writer. I've proven that LPNs and millennial nurses deserve a seat at the table. Most of all, I realize there is so much more for me.

I am now, in the next stage of my business. I have begun to implement quality assurance for long term care, home health, and nursing home facilities; charting education; and concierge writing services. As a millennial nurse, I often see and have experienced the gap between millennials and their coworkers. Therefore, I have implemented millennial diversity training and am constantly researching and implementing ways to balance the scales. I aspire to open an assisted living facility. I am currently in the research phase, with plans to launch within the next two years. Understanding the power of education, I am pursuing a Bachelor's in Healthcare Administration; upon completion, I plan to enroll in an accelerated Bachelor's of Science in Nursing program where a great deal of my career's focus will be education on healthcare disparities in underserved communities.

I am often asked what I would tell other nurses who are aspiring to become nurse entrepreneurs. My advice is simple and practical. Find out who you are and then discover who you'll be as a business owner. I suffered from depression, anxiety, and low self-esteem most of my life. I knew I could not take that with me into business. If I did, I would have a business full of those same qualities. I started working on myself and knew if I wanted to pour into other healthcare professionals' lives, I needed to be healed and whole. Owning a business or a brand is not as simple as having a name. Your brand needs to have an identity. You need to stick to that identity strictly out of the gate. If you want to be taken seriously, then you need to position yourself to be a key player with the movers and shakers in your industry. Hire professionals. Professional headshots and business cards are a must. Once your brand takes off, you will be asked to join panels, be a guest speaker, and etcetera. If you do not have a professional headshot, you won't be taken seriously. Professional headshots, a website, logos, and graphics are a minimal foundation for your brand.

Seek out consultants and/or mentors who have already accomplished what you are aspiring to accomplish. These people have been through the trials and tribulations and can help save you some mistakes, time, and money. FIND A MENTOR! You will need someone to talk to when things are not going the way you envisioned them. You need an unbiased expert to bounce ideas off and even to be critical when the time comes. There will be times that your family and friends won't understand your vision and they will discourage you. Having a mentor or someone with whom you can talk to in confidence will enable you to overcome those dark moments. Network makes your net worth. Networking has been the change I needed to get my brand where it is today. I am still fulfilling my mantra and I will continue to shed a little bit of light on whomever I encounter. Each day, I grab my lipstick and stethoscope and I have the mindset that, "Today is the day that my brand is going to change the world!"

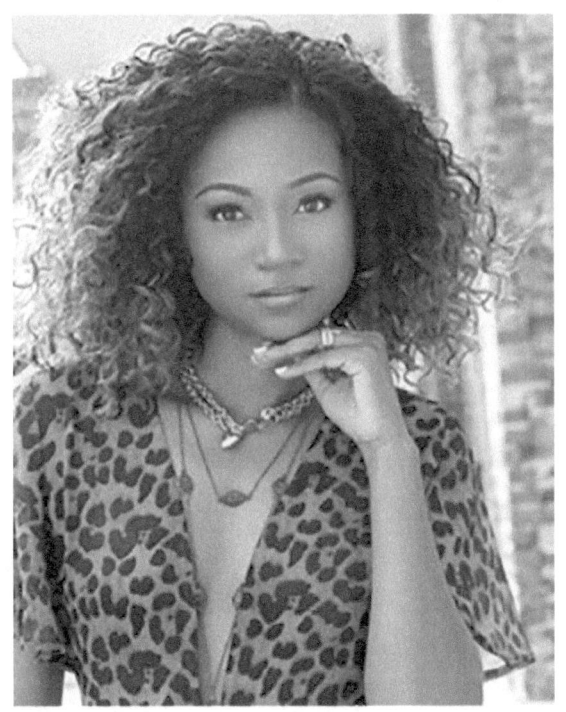

About the Author

Portia Wofford is a professional nurse with experiences in geriatrics, long term care, home and public health, care coordination and management, quality assurance, and patient education. Born in a small town in Alabama and raised by a single father, she learned at an early age how to care for others, which would serve her well in her nursing career. Wofford is the founder of *Your Nurse Connection,* conceived to bridge the gap between healthcare professionals and the community in which they serve through education, advocacy, empowerment, and support. Often being coined "The Millennial Nurse" Portia has landed roles as a contributing writer, published author, and healthcare content marketer. Offering millennial diversity training; quality assurance for long-term care, and nursing home facilities; and concierge writing services, this Generation Y thought leader is proving that millennial nurses deserve a seat at the table. Additionally, she is the mother of one son, a mentor, and has been deemed a fashionista, as she enjoys styling her family and friends.

To Connect With The Author:

Instagram: @yourNurseconnection

@lipstickandstethoscope

Facebook: Your Nurse Connection

Twitter: @Nurse_connect

Linkedin: Portia Wofford- The Millennial Nurse

Email: nurse1connection@gmail.com

Website: www.theNurseconnect.com

STEPPING INTO MY SEASON

Nicole Tyson-Ferguson, BSN, RN, CM/DN

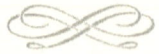

    Born to two working class parents, as a little girl I had a pretty decent life. Although I vaguely remember the details of my early childhood, photo albums and family stories painted pictures in my head. My grandmother would take me to church and made it her business to ensure that I would have a relationship with God. My mom worked for the government at the age of 19 and my father worked for a well-known vehicle manufacturing company until starting his own businesses. I was the first-born of my mom's three children, and the second of my father's two. I lived in the house with my mom and brothers, while my sister resided with our father and her mother. When you're a child, there are certain things you don't fully understand, and our blended family dynamics were not considered the norm. I didn't ask questions, nor did I answer them. My years as a teenager were a little complicated and somewhat difficult. For one, I had to babysit my brothers while my mom worked, and I was resentful for that.

    My mother was super strict; I couldn't do anything or go anywhere. All I wanted to do was be a normal teenager and hang out with my friends. Most of the time I was angry, confused, and would find myself crying a lot. One summer I was stuck in the house babysitting and decided to run away just to go to a neighborhood pool. As a result, I received one of the worst butt whoopings of my life. At this time, it was very easy to succumb to peer pressure and the desire to fit in. I was lacking information needed to survive in the real world because back then, a lot of parents didn't talk to their children. It wasn't until I got to middle school that I learned about sex education. Even though my mother drove me to and from school, I still managed to hook school and cut class. I lived this whole other life of lying and sneaking around. It seemed like I had to if I wanted one ounce of happiness. Or at least that's what I thought. Even though my decisions weren't smart ones, I had some fun and a little bit of freedom.

After being suspended from school, one of my friend's uncles pretended to be a family member and had me reinstated. My parents never knew and had they known, I would have been in big trouble. What I didn't realize until later was that they really cared, hence the reason why I wasn't allowed to do whatever I wanted. I had a lot of friends who could, and that made me think my life was just awful. The summer before high school I was hanging out with my cousin and met an older guy. I was 14 and he was 17. I'm pretty sure I lied about my age because by then I had become a pro. We talked on the phone a few times, but of course I had to sneak and do that. I joined the high school's cheerleading squad and used practice as an excuse to spend time with him. He introduced me to a totally different environment than what I was used to. I became pregnant at 15, and when my mother found out she hit the roof. I remember being scared and the constant smacks and yelling. We got in the car and drove to New York during a snowstorm to terminate the pregnancy. When we arrived, she took one look at the medical facility's conditions, and decided not to force me to proceed with the procedure.

The moment anyone tries to demean or degrade you in any way, you must know how great you are. Nobody would bother to beat you down if you were not a threat."
    Cicely Tyson

    We headed back home, and I was going to have a baby. How in the world could a baby raise a baby? I mean I knew a few young girls with babies, but not many. As sick as it may sound, having a baby seemed like the "in thing." Maybe this would be my opportunity to love someone and have them truly love me. I received a lot of backlash, negativity, and assassination of my character. Believe it or not, it was mainly family that had so much to say. I continued going to school and worked at a few fast food restaurants. On July 1, 1989, I gave birth to my first daughter. I was young, confused, and literally unable to process what was happening in my life. Gullible and naïve, you couldn't convince me that the baby's father, myself, and our little baby weren't a family. Having a child didn't change a thing because my mother was still strict and now I had even more responsibilities. Sometimes I felt like I was in prison and most of the time I was miserable. I swear I hated my life. My mother worked night shift and watched my daughter during the day so that I could go to school. Depending on her mood, I sometimes engaged in activities such as parties and skating on the weekends.

    I had a close relationship with my daughter's paternal family, but even as a young mother I was over protective and would not leave my daughter with anyone other than my mother. Two years later, on July 16, 1991, my second daughter was born. It was way too much!!!! She cried all day and night.

She just wouldn't stop crying at all. I was exhausted!! Although I can't place the blame on anyone but myself, lack of knowledge played a major role in me becoming a teenage parent. As much as I loved my daughters, I have always regretted not making better choices. Not giving myself enough time to grow and the ability to properly provide for them. Now I'm 18 with two kids, living in my mother's house in one room. Both of my parents supported us and gave as much help as humanly possible. Others gossiped, looked down on me, and judged my situation. What I did notice was that those same ones never offered any help or an encouraging word. I stayed in school, completed summer school, and eventually graduated. Yes, the girl with the two kids earned a high school diploma. With no life plan in order and college being the furthest thing from my mind, I was lost.

I had no dreams or goals, but what I did know was that I wanted to just live, feel free, and have fun. I enrolled in a six-month Certified Nursing Assistant certification program. After completion of the course, I took a position at a nursing home in Baltimore County. At the time, cloth diapers were used for incontinent patients. My least favorite part of the job was using the water hose to remove the feces from those diapers. I worked there for six months and after one of the patients had a bowel movement on my shoes, I resigned. That whole nursing home atmosphere was dark, smelly, and depressing.

> "It's not the load that breaks you down, it's the way you carry it."
> Lena Horne

Maybe I wasn't mature enough, but I could no longer do it. One of my girlfriends had an aunt and two older friends that worked for a company catering to the developmentally disabled. They helped me get a position there. I liked my job because it was easy, flexible, the clients were a joy to be around, and I worked with some familiar faces. My daughters' father had spent time in and out of jail and became addicted to drugs. We fought all the time and I kept it hidden from my parents, especially my father. Whenever he was able, he would help me and the girls; but for the most part, I was on my own.

I did whatever was necessary to make sure those little girls were taken care of and I mean WHATEVER!!! A lot of those things in which I'm not proud. Being involved in situations where I could have lost my life or faced incarceration is a chilling understatement. Associating myself with toxic people and engaging in unhealthy relationships, I was in way over my head. As the saying goes, "God looks out for fools and babies." Well he most definitely kept this fool covered. As I look back at my life, I know he wasn't finished with me yet and there was work to be done. One morning while transporting some clients in the company van, one of the clients yanked my ponytail and I lost control of the wheel. I woke up in the hospital bruised and banged up. From what I was told the van flipped over and was inches away from going over an embankment. My face was cut up pretty bad, to the point

> "No matter what accomplishments you make, somebody helped you."
> Althea Gibson

that my daughters were afraid to come near me. I healed well, but it was apparent that I would not be returning to work. In 1995, I packed up my girls and we moved into our own place. I didn't have one piece of furniture, just a truck full of toys and clothes. I had no permanent employment but was receiving some government assistance and doing agency work here and there.

My mother was against the move and my father was furious, so furious that he cut me off for a few months. This decision probably wasn't the best choice; but in my mind, I was thinking this would be an opportunity for me to gain my independence. Once again, I gave people something to talk about. I did that quite often. Sarcasm and criticism came from those who should have wanted the best for me and truthfully weren't in great positions themselves. I felt as if many wanted to see me fail. Of course, I didn't have it all figured out but I was going to try my best. With two kids, I definitely needed my own space. At some point, I kind of felt like my mother was enabling me. Let's just say that if I didn't take the initiative to venture out on my own she would have been okay with us staying with her forever. I love her for that, but I needed to start blooming into the woman I would become sooner than later. If things didn't work out I knew I could go back home, but I was going to do everything in my power not to.

A few months after we moved from the city, my daughters lost their father to street violence. They were too young to fully understand, and I was sad and full of guilt. I felt like I had snatched his family away and just left him in those streets. We had stopped seeing one another awhile before the tragedy; and the truth of the matter was that we were moving in opposite directions. I wanted better opportunities and education for my kids and never wanted to be stuck without options. I started applying for jobs at inner city hospitals and finally landed a position. My new job was in Downtown Baltimore; I didn't have a car and we lived in Rosedale, Maryland. It was no surprise when my mother came to the rescue - talk about a living angel here on earth. I would catch the bus to the hospital; she would meet me there to pick up my daughters, keep them overnight, pick me up in the morning, and drive us home. We did this same routine for a while until her work schedule changed. Living that far of a distance kept me out of the mix, but also helped open my eyes a lot.

It was so hard getting help when I needed it. Although it was extremely challenging, eventually I found a babysitter in the neighborhood to keep the girls overnight. I was doing better, and my father and I made amends. He bought me a car and things got a little easier. One September while riding home, the city and its surrounding counties experienced some rain fall and flooding. My car was stuck under a bridge of rising water and I was trapped inside. Imagine how grateful I was when two men came over and rescued me from the car to safety? That could have been a total catastrophe, especially since I could not swim. Due to the water damage, the car was totaled. I just could not catch a break. Taking so many steps forward, only to go backwards. The car was in my father's name, so the plan was for him to find me another one. We eventually went to a car auction and purchased a vehicle. Weeks had passed, frustration set in, and still no car. To this day, I'm not quite sure what happened, but I remember having a screaming match with my father via telephone. I was at my mother's house and my father came banging on the door. I was terrified so there was no way I was opening that door. He had never laid a hand on me ever, but I couldn't take any chances. My mouth messed that up and I was cut off yet again!!! This was really starting to get old.

My aggressiveness, attitude, and inability to control my emotions would always get the best of me. I reached out to my grandfather and he purchased a car for me. My cousin agreed to put the car in her name and that went smoothly until I had difficulties keeping up with the insurance payments. I was struggling more than ever this time around. For some reason, things would not get right. I was responsible for two children and bills; the money just wasn't adding up. The funny thing is that I was never able to get assistance with housing, vouchers, modified rent, etc. If you worked, the government had nothing for you. Talk about humiliating, once my cousin had to send her husband to my house with sanitary supplies. Every now and then I had a few friends that helped me out when possible, but nothing was consistent. Realistically no one owed me a thing. I needed to figure out some things and quickly. In December of 1996, I found out that I was pregnant. Why in the world would I even consider having another child knowing damned well I was struggling and could barely take care of the ones I already had? To this day, I still can't answer that question, and am clueless as to my what I was thinking back then.

> "My mission in life is not merely to survive, but to thrive, and to do so with some passion, some humor, and some style."
> Maya Angelou

By the spring of the following year, the girls and I moved into a more reasonable apartment and the new baby would be coming late summer. On August 20, 1997, my son was born. I was 24 and a little more mature as far as parenting was concerned. It was extremely difficult to find after-hour childcare for a newborn, let alone three kids. The term village truly kicked in this time around. I had aunts, cousins, and friends helping me out when feasible. Eventually, poor attendance led to termination from my job. It was time to begin my employment search again. I returned to the agency for assignments here and there. A few days after my son's first birthday, I accepted a position as a Surgical Technologist on a Labor and Delivery unit. This was a dream job where I would truly grow, acquire most of my skills, and be surrounded by a group of empowering women. It's amazing how God opens doors for you because I had a CNA certification and knew nothing about being a Surgical Technologist. Technically, I didn't even qualify for the position; but somehow, I was grandfathered in and trained.

The nurses with whom I worked were smart and they knew their stuff. They were always teaching me things, sharing information, and serving as positive role models. We were like one big family and I was the baby with babies. I'll never forget the words said to me by one nurse, "Don't you ever let me hear you say you don't know how to do anything". She taught me how to start an IV with an orange, now imagine that? I practiced hard and over the years became one of the best phlebotomists on our unit. I would even travel to other units to assist their staff with difficult sticks. This was a great place to work. I was happy, fulfilled, and making good money. In 2001, I started taking prerequisite courses at a local community college with hopes of getting accepted into their nursing program. As life happened, I took classes, passed, failed, stopped going, and started again. I did this on and off for about nine years. I worked, took care of my children, traveled, and partied. Life was good (from my clueless perspective) and I was living.

In 2004, one of my close male friends whom I dated for eight years was involved in a traumatic, life changing accident. After talking things over with my daughters, I stepped up to aid in his road to recovery. The plan was for him to stay with us until he healed and was back on his feet. The next thing I knew we were in a fully disclosed, mutual relationship. It kind of just happened and neither of us saw it coming. Although it was nice being in a real relationship and having a man around the house, it was a challenge as well. I was used to being independent and he was used to being in a male dominant role. We were having major power struggles, but he was what I needed and vice versa.

Things were going great and in 2006 we purchased our first home. Two years later, I resigned from my job and accepted a position at another facility closer to my home, offering a more generous salary. Let's just say, "the grass is not always greener on the other side." The Surgical Technologists at this facility were much older than me and had been there for years. I wanted to finish school and because they were set in

> *"I've come to believe that each of us has a personal calling that's as unique as a fingerprint – and that the best way to succeed is to discover what you love and then find a way to offer it to others in the form of service, working hard, and allowing the energy of the universe to lead you."*
> Oprah Winfrey

their ways, my school schedule could not be accommodated. I continued there for about two years and took what courses I could. The finish line was getting closer; I could see it, but I was having a hard time reaching it. Both of my daughters had graduated high school and my son was accepted into a Magnet High School. They lived pretty good lives, didn't want for anything, and had lots of support. I did pretty well raising three intelligent, well-mannered children. In January 2010 I was accepted into Coppin State University's nursing program. After a two-year engagement, in September I was married via a private ceremony at Magen's Bay in the U.S. Virgin Islands. In December of that same year, I was terminated from my job and four months later returned to my previous place of employment. As school became more intense and time consuming, I adjusted my work schedule from full time to part time. I received a tremendous amount of support and encouragement from my co-workers and friends. For the first time, I had a good feeling about my future. I've always had a head full of ideas but trouble executing them.

My husband and I collaborated and formed a real estate investment company. Business was booming but certain aspects of it seemed more frustrating than beneficial. It was 2014 and with hard work and perseverance, I was about to graduate with a Bachelor of Science in Nursing. The love I was shown was overwhelming. I remember walking out of my pinning ceremony and seeing several of my friends and family members in tears. That's when you know it's real. The people who know your journey and witnessed your struggles and sacrifices. People that are genuinely happy for you. Graduation day came, went, and now it was time to prepare to sit for the NCLEX. Even thinking about it gives me a headache. Talk about a stressful time. To my surprise, after three attempts and $1,400 later, I passed the NCLEX and was officially a Registered Nurse. Thank You Lord!!!! Career wise, I felt compelled to be a Labor and Delivery nurse because I had worked in the area for so long. I was interested in the Operating Room as well. While I was running out of options at my current place of employment I decided to cut my ties and find my way.

I took a position as a Labor and Delivery nurse at another facility but really did not feel comfortable with the staffing shortage nor the support during emergency situations. Besides, I worked hard for this license not to mention the time it took me to obtain it. Malpractice suits were occurring more frequently, and I wasn't willing to take a risk. I resigned from that position and leaped at the chance to work in the Operating Room. Although I liked this change, for some reason I felt unfulfilled. Being a blood and guts type of girl, I needed adrenalin rushing excitement which lead me to my next move and one of my best moves to date the Trauma Operating Room. When I did share time there, I knew I belonged. I felt at home. From gunshot wounds, stabbings, motor vehicle accidents, amputations, necrotizing fasciitis, touching a brain, holding a skull in my hands, removing organs from a donor, to cracking a chest open, I was finally fulfilled!!! I had found my passion. In the beginning, things weren't easy by far and I experienced some rough days. Actually, I still do today. Surrounded daily by death and traumatic situations can take a toll on you mentally. The go getter in me stood tall and pushed through. There is no better feeling than saving lives and learning while doing so.

As I reflect, I remember the moment I became interested in becoming a nurse. I was working for an agency as a sitter and my patient's nurse was a few years older than me. Impressed by her stature, I began asking her tons of questions. The entire time I was thinking to myself, "I can be a nurse." My great grandmother was in the nursing field; it's quite possible that observing her nurture and care for others may have influenced me as well. She lived well, traveled, and took care of her family. I admired her and although others may not have known, I was watching and taking mental notes. For those looking to pursue a career in nursing or start a business, I would strongly advise you to go for it. There is no such thing as too young or too old. It doesn't matter how long it takes, but what does matter is that you stick with it. Nothing in life comes easy. If you believe it, you can achieve it. More importantly, you should be passionate about your craft and not in it for the sole purpose of financial gain. The goals you set for yourself should never be impacted by anyone else's opinions or doubts. You only get one life, so believe me, you want to make it count. Having been a nursepreneur for only a short time, I can say I enjoy the freedom and benefits of working for myself and making my own rules.

Some of the most important things I've learned through experience and networking with other entrepreneurs:

- The importance of good planning and organizational skills.
- Always provide impeccable customer service.
- Try creating a new market instead of existing within.
- Be flexible, unpredictable, and consistent.
- Investing in macro goals should be one of your biggest commitments.
- Stand behind your brand without compromising the purpose and integrity of your business.
- Have realistic expectations of profit and loss.

> "Once you know who you are, you don't have to worry anymore."
> Nikki Giovanni

It made sense to start a business that would reflect my passion for healthcare. A business that would allow me to offer a variety of services. I was scared with tons of negative thoughts running through my mind, especially since I had a prior business fail. What if it doesn't work out? What if I'm wasting my money? What if I don't get any clients? The list goes on and on. I noticed that I was my worst critic and at times I didn't give myself enough credit. Also, I needed to be mindful of sharing too much information. Everyone doesn't need to know your every move. I was told I had no patience and I expected things to happen overnight. The minute I stepped back, prayed, and got rid of those negative seeds of doubt, the calls started coming and the clients started to appear. Having been certified as a Delegating Nurse for less than a year, my clientele is steadily growing day by day. The mind of an entrepreneur is one that is always racing, strategizing, and exploring new business ventures. While I am planning to return to school to obtain a Master's degree as well as purchase commercial real estate sometime in the near future. The success of my current businesses takes precedence. My latest project is Generation 5 Healthcare, Inc., a corporation offering direct care support services to the developmentally disabled, along with health care training to its employees and the general population. My overall goal is to provide alternative living units, transportation services, and a day habilitation program. Clients will receive assistance with their day to day transitions through life in safe, family-oriented environments. Trusting the process, I am patiently awaiting licensure and optimistic about each and every one of my future endeavors. What's for me is for me!!

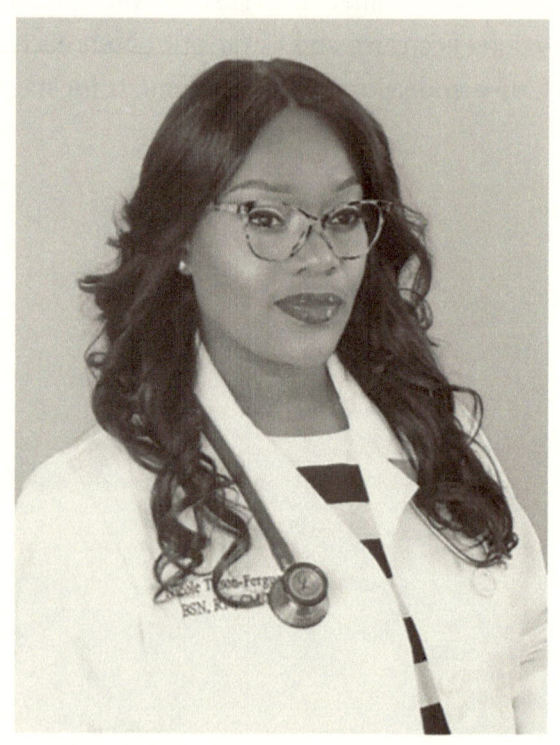

About the Author

Having assumed the role of caretaker at a very young age, it was no secret that Nicole Tyson-Ferguson would excel as a compassionate nurse. As a teen mom, Nicole faced obstacle after obstacle, but steered the course to provide a legacy for her family. Beginning her healthcare career as a CNA, and working as a Surgical Technologist for over 17 years, Nicole received her Bachelor of Science degree in Nursing from Coppin State University in Baltimore, Maryland. Today, just four years shy of graduation, Nicole is a skilled nurse in the specialty areas of Labor and Delivery, General Operating Room, and Trauma Operating Room. She is a certified instructor for Advanced Cardiac Life Support, Cardiopulmonary Resuscitation, and the Medication Technician Training Program. Nicole is also co-owner of a real estate investment company and Delegating Nurse for several Assisted Living facilities throughout the Baltimore Metropolitan area. The most important roles fulfilled by Nicole include wife, mother, grandmother, and ambitious entrepreneur. In her pastime, Nicole enjoys divulging in shopping, traveling, singing, dancing, and spending time with family and friends. Even with all the hats Nicole wears, she continuously feels she is not doing enough to help others. Her need to become more involved with the behavioral health community led her to form Generation 5 Healthcare, Inc. Nicole enacts her vision to create an environment which offers various support programs in family-oriented settings by catering to the needs of the developmentally disabled.

To Contact The author:

Email: nursenikki14@verizon.net

Facebook: Nicole Tyson-Ferguson

Instagram: @nursenikki14

CENTERED BEAUTY: NEVER STOP DREAMING

Audrey Lovings-Clark, BSN, RN

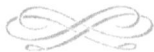

Growing up in a small town by the name of La Marque, Texas, there were not very many role models and overachievers. Families such as mine were akin to television shows such as the Jefferson's and the theme song *"Moving on Up."* My family and I found ourselves "moving on up" when we were blessed with the opportunity to move out of Galveston, Texas. The part of town in which we lived in was (more or less) considered "the ghetto", so theoretically the move meant we were a bit more financially stable than the average family; however, greatness always seemed to run the other way. Over the years, I looked on in amazement while my mom, who was a nurse, and my dad, a pipe fitter, worked hard to provide for our family. When I use the word "family", I am referring to more than just my immediate family. Family included more than just those that lived under our roof permanently. One of the first aha moments for me was coming to the realization that my parents put in a ton of hard work and long hours; however, there were never any conversations with us about dreams and goals.

Being the youngest child in the family, with an older sister and brother, afforded me the opportunity to learn from their mistakes; however, some genetics and socializations were inbred. As I reflect on my childhood, we seemed to "just do it". Not like Nike though. As I look back, I cannot recall any deep conversations whatsoever about dreams and goals. That was very peculiar because my sister was pretty much a genius; she had so much drive she could have become our first female president if she aspired to.

As I grew older, one of the statements I would hear most often was, "You are going to college." At times, I felt as though the thought of me going to college was my parents last bit of hope. Especially since neither of my siblings went to college right after high school. Work, work, and more work was all I witnessed. Diligently, both parents worked day and night to provide a better life for us. My siblings and I developed an excellent work ethic because of my parents. I also acquired a burning desire for SUCCESS. The funny thing is, I had a strange feeling when I was younger that I could work hard and will myself to success. At an early age, I took a special interest in the art of styling hair and transforming women.

My sister took cosmetology courses during her high school years; she also did some modeling. Having the opportunity to watch my sister style hair, do makeup, and just seeing her sense of fashion was a huge catalyst in my love for cosmetology. We were also lucky enough to have our childhood hairdresser live directly across the street. I was amazed and inspired as I watched women being transformed. They would drive up and walk into her home appearing to lack self-confidence but would leave with a renewed sense of self. That meant the world to me and it was one of my biggest muses.

That ignited me to start my own business, which was opening a hair salon in my mother's kitchen as well as in my bedroom. The first name I gave my salon was Yahne's Jazzy Connections. Back then, I had a dream of helping women transform and build their self-confidence. Living in a small town exposed me to tons of women with low self-esteem and insecurities. It was truly satisfying just knowing I played a part in helping to alleviate this; not to mention, the income I generated in high school enabled me to help my parents save money on my school clothes. It also afforded me the opportunity to buy myself nice things. This was beyond rewarding, and it gave me a sense of inner joy and accomplishment. The sense of independence I felt was incomparable. It was gratifying to know I could help alleviate some of my parents' stressors after witnessing their blood, sweat, and tears.

During my senior year at La Marque High School, my business really started to grow; and the conversations were nondirectional in reference to goals and dreams. I was pretty much going through the motions and trying to make a name for myself as a great "kitchen beautician". Young girls and their mothers would line up and sit in my room in front of the mirror on the door of my closet, getting the latest trendy hairdo for a fraction of the cost. Before I knew it, the last semester of school had arrived, which meant it was crunch time for me. Many of my classmates were committing to colleges and some were showing off multiple acceptance letters. Honestly, the thought of going to college out of state did not appeal to me at all, so I was in limbo trying to search for a college to attend. I took the SAT test and did well; however, no schools were contacting me. Lamar University was on the radar as a great school that was not too close to home, but also not too far away. I applied and got accepted.

Finally, I found myself with answers to the questions that had been on "repeat and replay" for quite some time. "What college are you going too?" "What are you majoring in?" I was finally positioned to answer those questions with great confidence and assurance. Now, I could answer them without blinking an eye, "Lamar University and I am majoring in Psychology." But deep down within my core, I wanted to be a beautician and own my own salon. I even had the first name for my salon all picked out; it was Yahne's Jazzy Connections. I knew my acceptance letter to Lamar University had pretty much eased the tension for my parents and had silenced the phrase, "You are going to go to college." You see, for some strange reason, my parents felt as if college was the only option for me. Because I was a child that always followed my parents' orders, off to college I went! At that point, I and those in my inner circle desperately needed an intervention.

Once I arrived at college, my sense of style and unique hairstyle changes opened the opportunity for my hair business. Two weeks after I started college, my life suffered a major blow. I recall walking into my dorm room after class one day and seeing a note on the door that read, "Please call home, family emergency!!!" It felt as if my heart had stopped beating as I was being transported to the airport and flown to Galveston from Beaumont, Texas. I learned that my dad had been involved in a deadly accident at the chemical plant where he was employed. He had suffered burns over 80% of his body. Thankfully, my dad pulled through and survived; however, at that moment, I felt as though my emotions were completely numb. Unfortunately, it stayed that way for many years.

As I reflect on that dark time, I now realize that a part of my brain (amygdala) had been figuratively lacerated. I was emotionally dead for at least two decades. I had no other alternative but to remain strong and literally go through the motions daily. I had to swallow and embrace the fact that my dad - my hero and the man that I had always looked up to - would never be the same again. If you've never been in my shoes, it's hard to imagine the pain that a "daddy's girl" feels while watching him be reduced to infancy for months and months. The strength that my mother displayed as his caregiver was unfathomable. It was the first of many instances that I could assist in the care of a loved one. It's true what they say, "What does not kill you will make you stronger". Albeit you may be emotionally withdrawn, but nevertheless stronger. I so wanted to return home and help my mother care for my dad, but they both insisted that I stay in college and finish what I started.

The next few years continued to solidify and confirm that I was indeed an artist. My weekly hairstyle changes and trendy wardrobe made huge fashion statements. I was known around campus as the girl who styled hair and had a great eye for fashion. Styling hair was a great source of income for me while I was in college, and it also gave me the ability to connect with other women on campus. The community in Beaumont, Texas was awesome, and the residents were very genuine and down to earth. A year later, I decided to change my major from Psychology to Nursing. I was aware that nursing school would be quite challenging. Having pledged to become a member of the amazing Alpha Kappa Alpha Sorority Incorporated, it provided me with the tenacity needed to complete the task at hand. There is an old quote that states, "Excuses are tools upon which we build monuments of nothingness, and those who dwell upon them are seldom good for anything else." The bottom line is to stop making excuses and start making progress.

The work ethic that was instilled in me by my parents helped me to stay the course in nursing school. Becoming a nurse has been one of my most gratifying accomplishments yet. The journey became a bit easier for me as the semesters went by. It was then when I had an epiphany that I could achieve anything my heart desired. I knew deep within my core I had to finish nursing school. There were no other alternatives for me. I knew I had to become the first person in my family to graduate from a university. I was the last of three children, and I was expected to be the first college graduate. I also knew I had a younger cousin who looked up to me, and I wanted nothing more than for her to witness me accomplish my mission.

Surprisingly, there were many in the nursing program before me who had failed to pass the State Board Exam; therefore, the school began implementing exit exams to ensure a greater passing rate. It seemed I studied more in the last few months of college than I ever did during the entire program. I passed the State Board Exam on the initial attempt and then graduated. At that point, I was sort of bewildered about what the future held and what my next steps would be. School had been a long, rocky road for me; but it was beyond rewarding. The mere thought of nurturing and helping others to heal truly warmed my heart. It served as a good replacement for the sense of fulfillment that styling hair gave me.

To say I was proud to have followed in my mother's footsteps of becoming a nurse was a huge understatement! She was a Licensed Vocational Nurse, and I was officially a Registered Nurse. Ironically, I had no plan of action for which route I wanted to take in my new career. Many had plans of working in the Intensive Care Unit, Emergency Room, or

Labor & Delivery. On the other hand, I was still having inhibitions about working long, 12-hour days in the same building. I couldn't get past the thought of going into work before sunrise and getting off after sunset. I remember so vividly during my clinical rotation, being pressed for time because there were so many patients to tend to. I so wanted to give back rubs to patients if need be, but was not able to do so due to time constraints. I would also prefer to take my time and thoroughly instruct my patients who were being discharged about their orders and home medications. The fact that I had to rush when treating patients disturbed me ethically. It eventually created a mental barrier which deterred me from hospital nursing.

As I reflect, I am reminded of the twilight zone. Day to day, I had visions of varicose veins, worn down tennis shoes, body aches, and the mere agony of being overworked. That is what I witnessed every day, in every hallway and nurses' station. Inevitably, I developed an affinity for Community Health Nursing. The light bulb came on and I knew immediately I had finally found my happy place! I was excited about the opportunity to be able to teach my clients and ensure that the transition from hospital to home was a smooth one. Having nursing assistance experience enabled me to help them with their activities of daily living such as bathing and any other necessities.

For two decades, local health departments and home health agencies have been my area of interest and expertise. If we can envision it then we can become it! Networking is our greatest resource! Our brain is our biggest weapon! "As a man thinketh in his heart, so is he". We must learn to stop carrying baggage that we do not need. At one point in my life, I let go of my dreams; however, resilience, persistence, and focus kept my head above water. Approximately two years ago, there was an awakening - a birth story of sorts. The nurse in me decided to share brain space with the artist in me. If I truly believed all the motivational speakers to whom I had listened and their "you can do anything speeches", then I had to believe in myself fully. God was, is, and always will be on my side. Those on the outside looking in would probably look at me and think, "she always gets her way." Little do they know of the struggles and challenges that haunted me for two decades.

Divine intervention is what brought my dreams into fruition. God made it so clear that He even gave me a new name for my hair business - "Centered Beauty". He even gave me the scripture to govern my business and my life by, which was Philippians 4:6, "Don't worry about anything; instead, pray about everything." Centered Beauty, where beauty is well balanced, confident, and serene. The core of my company is centered around the beauty of a woman which starts on the inside. We specialize in custom hairpieces that help save women time and money, while enhancing their inner and outer beauty. If you look good, then you feel good; and if you feel good, you look good. Centered beauty takes a holistic approach toward beauty. As a nurse entrepreneur, I plan to further my education and become a Family Nurse Practitioner. I also aspire to expand Centered Beauty into a one-stop shop beauty and wellness center. The secret to success is to always follow your heart and relentlessly pursue your dreams. The sky is the limit, so reach for the stars!

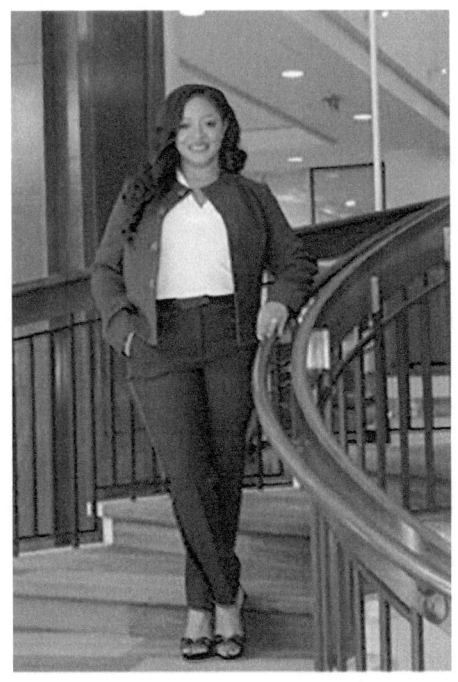

About the Author

Driven by passion to help others, Audrey Lovings-Clark strives for greater successes in areas that she not only loves but also finds joy in sharing her creative talents and skill. Twenty years ago, she graduated from Lamar University (Beaumont, Texas) with a Bachelor of Science in Nursing. To further become involved and committed to sisterhood and community service, she became a member of Alpha Kappa Alpha Sorority Incorporated in the Fall of 1993. Her nursing career started in Community Health due to a passion and love for teaching and assisting clients in the home environment. Public Health Nurse,

Program Manager, Director of Nurses in Home Health, Nurse Case Manager, and Nurse Coordinator are the positions she has served in during her twenty-year nursing career. She also adores making women feel beautiful and exceptional, which led to her studying Cosmetology at Royal Beauty Careers. For two years, she has been licensed to perform the passion that God deposited into her as a child. Her aim is not only to help women feel wonderful and fierce on the outside, but to also develop within them a sense of wonder and worth unmatched by all the forces and struggles in the world that pull women down and apart. Her goal is to have a one-stop shop for Women's Wellness and Beauty Enhancements. Her company, Centered Beauty, was developed as a result which specializes in non-surgical hair replacement (custom units, wigs) and all healthy hair care services. Audrey is the wife of a loving husband of 11 years with whom she has two sons, ages 8 and 20.

To Contact The Author:

Instagram – @centered_beauty

Facebook – Audrey Lovings-Clark

Periscope – AudreyLovings-Clark

centeredbeauty@gmail.com

EMPIRE STATE OF MIND

Freda Watson

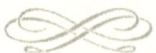

I was born and raised in Providence Rhode Island. As a child, I was taken away from my mother and placed in foster care, because some family members thought she was too young to raise me and my brother. Subsequently, they told lies until they succeeded to get us taken away from her. My mother fought hard and never gave up on getting me back. I watched her go through the worst trials and tribulations. My mother was a young parent trying to find her way. Even though she didn't always know what to do as a parent, she tried her best. I and my brother's father were in prison serving ninety-nine years for murder, so my mother had no help. She worked small jobs and we lived in a shelter for a little while until we moved into Hartford Projects. While growing up in the projects, I was exposed to drugs, alcohol, guns, and crime. However, we didn't stay that long in the projects. We ended up going to live with my auntie Carolyn who was a Registered Nurse.

While living with my auntie Carolyn, I was curious about what a nurse did, so I would follow her around and ask a thousand questions about what a nurse was. One day I watched her give herself a shot and I asked: "why are you doing that?" She would say "I'm a diabetic." I didn't know what that meant at the time. My auntie didn't mind at all and would answer all my questions. My auntie Carolyn would tell me to go get one of her many medical books off the shelf. She explained to me what a diabetic was and how important it was to give herself shots. I would also spend a lot of time with my other auntie, Loretta, who also was a Registered Nurse. I would sometimes go to her job with her and see all her patients. I wanted to help, but I couldn't because I was too young. Spending all this time and learning so much from my aunts, made me want to care for others.

One summer in the 80's, my mother thought it would be a good idea for me to go stay the summer with my auntie in Georgia. Little did she know that would change my life forever. I ended up staying to go to elementary school that year. One day I missed the bus and I had to stay home. All my cousins had already left for school and the only person left in the house was my auntie's boyfriend. He took me to my auntie's room and raped me. I was only nine years old when my auntie's boyfriend raped me, and I never told anybody until I got in my late twenties. I left Georgia when school was over and went back to Rhode Island. I was glad that my nightmare was over in Georgia. Subsequently, I went back home with my mother who was pregnant with my sister. I met her boyfriend who I grew up with some of his family. He was a nice guy at the time until one day he decided to start molesting me at the age of eleven, until I was sixteen.

The molesting stopped when my mother finally caught him coming out my room late one night. I got up the next morning and went to school. When I came back home he was gone for good. I never told, because he was the breadwinner in the house and my mother never really worked. I was afraid if I told he would go to jail and my mother wouldn't have any money to take care of me and my little sisters. I was determined not to let this break me down mentally, although I was physically and mentally abused most my life.

I carried on the rest of my teenage life as if nothing happened, then the shocker of my life came when I found out I was pregnant with my son at 17 years old. A baby? What am I going to do with a baby? I wanted to own a daycare and take care of babies, not have one so soon. Well, I had my son and I knew I really had to do something then. I had all these goals and visions that I wanted to accomplish. As time went by, I decided to create a vision board that I sat at the end of my bed. It was the last thing I saw when I went to sleep and the first thing I saw when I woke up.

My vision board kept me motivated and gave me a reason not to give up on my dreams and aspirations. I accomplished getting my Georgia State early childhood license to open a daycare in 2010. I had so many bumps in the road with trying to get my business going well, but I kept pushing until one day my auntie, Victoria, said to me " don't force it, if it's meant to be it will be, God, knows best." Consequently, I put that on hold, but I refused to give up on my passion to help people.

I would think to myself "there's got to be another way I can help make a difference in someone's life." I would do private duty nursing. This entailed me going to houses assisting the elderly with the quality care that they needed. I would also go to my great-grandmother's house, who was 100 years old at the time. My mother was her caretaker and she never could find the extra help she needed with caring for my great-grandmother. I would hear her say " I can't do this all by myself." It was hard finding good nurses to come sit with my great-grandmother.

My sister's, my cousin, and I would do all we could to assist my mother with my great-grandmother. This influenced my decision to take $500 and open my first Home Care Business called "Sincere Home Care, LLC" in Brunswick Georgia. My great-grandmother, who I'm named after her only child, was a significant influence on me wanting to start a senior caregiving business. She was an independent lady and my mentor when I was younger. Later she relied on the family for various things such as toileting, bathing, preparing her meals, going to the store, and getting her out of bed. This is when I realized how much my great-grandmother really needed us and I was glad that I could be there to help her during her time of need. After she passed away, I thought about other seniors who may be facing the same or similar challenges as she did. When my great-grandmother passed away it made me think about family members who are overwhelmed by the various responsibilities and who are not fully equipped to deliver the kind of care their parents need. It made me want to start a new venture that specifically entails helping seniors with difficulties and those who seek guidance for taking on the responsibilities of planning and caring for their loved one. From being frustrated by my own experiences, I wanted to assist others.

I didn't know much about how to get my state license, but I didn't let that stop me. I researched countless days, nights, and hours, having to be up by 6 am, to get my children off to school and to be to work by 7 am, five days a week. This was because I was determined to find out all I could to get my Georgia home care license. I wanted to be able to hire the best Certified Nurse Assistants and nurses so that I can provide the best quality care to seniors in need.

I received my home care license in less than 60 days. I was so happy that I could now serve my community with the best quality care that they deserve. Subsequently, I now service several clients in 10 counties in the state of Georgia. I also employ several medical professionals who are great. They're caring, nurturing, and very reliable; and I could not ask for a better team to work with. Moreover, I can provide more for my children and my mother by having financial freedom. I can maintain my desired lifestyle without a regular paycheck now, all because I never gave up on my dreams when things got rough and I always put God first. Without God, none of this would be possible. I been doing private duty nursing since 2007 and I enjoyed it. I would sit with two or three clients a day and assist them with everyday life skills. I'm now working on my next business that will play a major part in the medical field as well. In essence, don't give up on your dreams no matter how hard it gets. Success is just around the corner. I will continue to do what I love and that's helping people.

I understand that the care I can facilitate through my industry and employees can be life-changing as well as life-saving for the individuals my industry serves. Some more reasons I have for becoming an entrepreneur is to have the opportunity to control my own destiny, the freedom to spend my time doing what I feel is important, and the opportunity to have a lasting legacy. Building a business that I am passionate about can impact the lives of my children because, I am leaving them something that I am proud of and that they can carry on. Another reason that I chose to become an entrepreneur is to contribute to society.

Building a senior care business can help me contribute to society because, I can create jobs, help others advance in life, help design better services to make customers happy, and help people in other ways. Being able to contribute to society will be very fulfilling for me as an entrepreneur. Moreover, knowing that I am making a positive difference in people's lives will make me feel proud of my business.

Tips For Other Nurses/People In General

If you hold certain characteristics it can be significant for you to consider a senior care industry. These characteristics include:

- You enjoy working with many types of people (e.g. patients, families, physicians, insurers, and employees) on a daily basis.

- You can empathize with patients as well as their family members. This entails being caring and tailoring your solutions with the consideration of certain problems they may be facing.

- You can remain objective when problems arise.

- You are logical which entails being able to offer practical solutions.

- You are outgoing and assertive.

- You are patient.

- You are observant. This entails noticing if an individual's condition is changing.

Another tip is it is necessary to ask questions. There is a saying that there is no such thing as a dumb question. Questions are important because, there is a lot to learn in the nurse field and asking them can help you to avoid doing something incorrectly. Also, asking questions can help you to remember the information more accurately and longer. The next tip that I feel is crucial is to avoid rushing.

Rushing might seem like a good idea when trying to get caught up at work. However, rushing can lead to mistakes. Therefore, it is crucial to slow down instead of going faster when you are behind on work. A suggestion is to plan ahead and organize certain tasks that involve patient care. Organizing work tasks can be beneficial because, it can help you to be more efficient and do less rushing. Getting organized is crucial and can help you to provide better nursing care, group your tasks, and be able to slow down. The next tip that I feel is important is to keep learning. As an entrepreneur, there is no end to what we can learn. Therefore, we must keep learning in order to grow. Providing care to individuals entails being committed to a career-long process of learning. On the other hand, an important tip is to make sure you take time for yourself. This means time for family, friends, relaxation, travel, and hobbies.

Taking time for ourselves is momentous because, it can influence our well-being as well as our personal fulfillment. Subsequently, my next suggestion is for caregivers to understand that it is essential for us to be helpful. Being helpful means offering to pitch in, volunteering; and showing others that you are willing to help, approachable, and cooperative when things get complex. Moreover, being helpful to those in need can be a huge satisfaction. Next, I feel that listening to patients is important.

Listening to patients is necessary because, they know their bodies better than you do. This tip is noteworthy because, it will help you to not only fully engage with your patients, but to make better decisions and deliver better patient care. Likewise, a caregiver should have integrity and honesty with him or herself as well as others. Even though honesty is crucial in all careers, it is essential in caregiving.

Honesty is essential because, caregivers frequently deal with patients in difficult situations, handle sensitive materials, and closely rely on coworkers Consequently, caregivers should evaluate their integrity regularly, and always look for ways to improve. The last tip is to believe in yourself. This involves believing in your instincts. Instincts can be significant because, it can let us know something is wrong with a patient. Furthermore, a tip to entrepreneurs is you can be educated without the degrees and become a millionaire, the first year in the non- medical home care business.

The non-medical home care business is a billion-dollar business. People may make it seem like you must have degrees and money to be successful and try to discourage you from trying to make it in life. In fact, so many successful leaders do not have a college degree (e.g. Steve Jobs, Henry Ford, Rachael Ray, Ralph Lauren, Steven Spielberg, Bill Gates, Mark Zuckerberg, Coco Chanel, and Oprah Winfrey etc.). Also, there are essentials that must be done first to get your non-medical home care business started. However, these items should not cost you much, and the money that your business will generate should cover the expense. With research, effort, and time, you will be on your way to a successful homecare business.

Your Industry

My industry involves providing home health care to seniors; and helping seniors who have trouble with doing everyday activities. The industry will provide a combination of medical care (e.g. administering antibiotics, private nursing, and helping with rehabilitation) and non-medical care (e.g. fixing meals, helping with chores, bathing, remembering to take his or her medication, getting dressed, general house cleaning, transportation, general companionship, overnight care, and etc.). My market will be clients who are seniors and their families.

Being the owner of a senior care industry will entail me sending qualified and compassionate individuals out to assist seniors with their daily living tasks. In essence, I will perform as a referral service through locating reliable, cheerful, kind, and honest individuals to place in seniors' homes; either temporary or long-term. Services will be personalized to each individual's physical needs. This will include the installation of improvements (e.g. stair lifts, wheel chair ramps, and grab bars).

This industry will help seniors by satisfying or filling a real need through helping them lead more independent lives. It will also lift the burden from family members who are worried when caring for an elderly loved one. I will use my experience in caregiving as well as business skills to build a relevant agency. Some of the main skills that will be required for me to run this business will be creativity, business savvy, and the ability to hold a consistent customer base.

How Has Nursing Helped Shape Your Business?

Nursing is very helpful in shaping my business because, it gives me the ability to offer medically trained caregiving services such as:

- Medication set-up and/or administration
- Insulin injections
- Dressing changes

- Wound care
- Catheter care
- Colostomy or Ostomy care
- Skilled hospice support
- Diabetes care and treatment

Obstacles You Have Faced Being An Entrepreneur

One challenge that I have faced being an entrepreneur is decision-making. Being a new entrepreneur has required me making many decisions daily. From making big decisions to small ones I have found myself experiencing decision fatigue. This has been a learning experience which has showed me how crucial it is for me to be prepared for a new level of stress and be able to effectively cope with stress. The next challenge that I have faced is dealing with the unknown.

Dealing with the unknown has led me to ask myself how long will my business last and how profitable will my business be? There is no certain answer. Therefore, it is important for me to be prepared for anything. Certain challenges can be stressful; however, I can reduce the stress by understanding workplace stress cannot be eliminated; but the stress can be reduced by making it a priority to care for myself. This entails balancing life and implementing useful self-care strategies. Conversely, distinguishing from competition has been another challenge I have faced as an entrepreneur.

It is crucial for my agency to be competitive, by being able to stand apart from other senior home care agencies. This entails me analyzing the competitors to identify their strengths, weaknesses, service processes, and etc. Being competitive will help me to get noticed, create trust among people, and build reputation. Moreover, this involves me improving my activities along with providing more effective service to my clients. This has been challenging, but it has been a learning process and has helped me to aim towards creating my own strategy for my agency.

Why It Was All Worth It

Building my own business as an entrepreneur is worth it because it will help seniors and can be an invaluable service to them. Research has shown that in-home care for seniors has proven to be one of the most effective care solutions available to them today. Being an entrepreneur gives me the opportunity to really make a difference in someone's life. Elderly patients essentially need the services that my agency will provide. By assisting seniors with personal care, I am providing a vital service to my patients. This also enables me to be an advocate for them.

Being an advocate for my patients allows me to make sure that their needs are being effectively communicated and satisfied. Conversely, being able to provide support for those who need it most makes my business worth it. I feel a great joy from being able to help someone, by assisting with daily activities, who is unable to fully care for himself or herself. Also, making someone smile or making someone's life easier makes the hard work that comes with running my business worth it.

My business involves spending time with patients and this has a real impact on their lives. This helps me to make a difference in someone's life. Not only can I help to improve the quality of life for my clients, I can carry that knowledge with me always. It is challenging; however, it is worth it. A venture in helping others is worth it because, it is a mutually beneficial experience. Making this my life's work makes me happy because, I can help someone accomplish something that they may not have had the ability to do without my help. I feel that my venture is worth it for various reasons. Other than supporting an individual or advocating on their behalf, the genuine appreciation that I receive from some clients is a great reminder of why I chose a venture in helping seniors.

My heart and mind are continuously opened to how I can grow, learn, and improve with each day that I work with seniors. I feel fortunate that each day I can help others and I learn so much from the people I work with. Therefore, I am challenged to learn on a daily basis. Knowing that I helped change someone's life circumstances in a better way is rewarding. It is rewarding when an individual tells me how much I have helped them. Making a positive difference in someone's life is worth it. Caregiving is something that I am passionate about, so I enjoy giving some of my time to this cause. It leaves me feeling not only rewarded but fulfilled. Moreover, caregiving is exciting because, each day is different, and you never know what is going to happen next. This means that I must solve problems, make effective decisions, and stay on my toes. On the other hand, caregiving allows me to build connections and get to know clients on a personal level.

Building connections and getting to know clients are two reasons why I love being a caregiver. Each special moment that I have with my clients makes me remember certain moments that I had with my great-grandmother. Working in my industry is not just a career to me, it is my calling. I have no doubt that working in a caregiving industry is in my nature because, I want to help elder individuals and I consider myself a very caring person. Also, my personal experiences have led me to fall into working in the caregiving field. A few benefits of working in my industry are:

- I can make a difference in the lives of my clients as well as their families. This involves building personal relationships and enhancing an individual's quality of life. This gives me a sense of accomplishment.

- I can provide companionship and social interaction to those who may need it. This can be personally rewarding.

- I have the ease of a flexible schedule.

- My venture can make life more manageable for my clients.

- I can help clients remain comfortable and safe at home.

- I have the opportunity for professional development and steady growth.

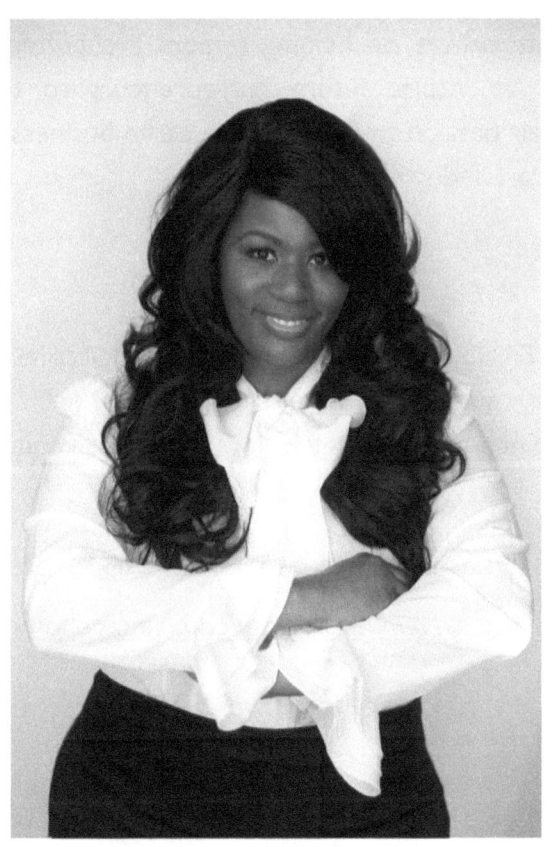

About the Author

Freda Watson is the CEO/Founder of Sincere Home Care, LLC. Her love and caring nature for people along with helping others is the reason she joined the Healthcare and Childcare Industry. Her dedication and experience with caring for elderly patients and children inspired her to open Sincere Home Care,

LLC. She is currently working on other medical endeavors to help educate others on helping seniors live better lives. She too hopes to inspire future entrepreneurs to be able to develop their passion to become successful business owners in the Healthcare Industry.

To Contact The Author:

Email: empirestateofmindset@gmail.com, sincerecareathome@gmail.com, or sincerehealthcaretrainingsolut@gmail.com

Website: sincerecareathome.com

Facebook: @sincerehomecarellc and @empirestateofmind18

Instagram: https://www.instagram.com/sincerehomecare912/

BEDSIDE TO BOSSTRESS

By: Drumeka Rollerson, BSN, RN

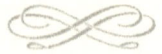

When I was initially asked to contribute to this anthology, I wondered how I could possibly make the time. Between being a mother, a wife, a nurse, and an entrepreneur I often believe twenty-four hours will never be enough time to accomplish my daily tasks; however, I am always honored and humbled anytime God gives me the opportunity to make His name great. Consequently, once I reevaluated the importance of giving God the glory in everything I do, this task was no longer about making time but *this* is about "the time(s)" My life is filled with undeniable God-Moments; these are the periods in my life that God proved *He* is my source, my guide, my strength, my keeper, my protector and the very reason I have committed to this literary work for this great cause. My journey of becoming a nurse and an independent entrepreneur is nothing short of God's awesomeness. Allow this abbreviated portion of "my story" [but God's glory] to encourage you, ignite a fire of determination within you, and help you understand and know that nothing is impossible [with God]. We have the ability to be greater than GREAT; and our greatness lies in our adamancy to overcome fear, be purpose driven [personally and interpersonally], and surround ourselves with like-minded people!

Anytime our destiny is filled with greatness, it seems that turbulent trials are inevitable; it is almost as if a story of tragedies and triumphs are expected. However, I understand all tragedies do not end in triumph and all triumphs are not rooted in tragedy. Fortunately, God allowed every trial in my life to develop me into the person I am now and the person I will become [we are continually evolving and being perfected].

I was raised by my mom and grandmother; I never really knew my father. My parents were teenagers when I was born. My dad was never a consistent or reliable presence in my life. I received sporadic phone calls from him - once every three to five years. I can remember my mom and I living in different housing projects and apartments as she did her best to work and provide for me at such a young age. As an adolescent, I can vividly recall the heartbreak I felt every time my father failed to keep his word and visit me. My parents were only fifteen years old when they became parents. Inevitably, my grandmother was an unwavering constancy in my life. I shudder at the thought of my existence, if she were not a part of my life. I know her prayers and love have kept me. We did not have much money but the love we shared was plentiful and made me understand what it truly meant to *be valued*. I recall my grandmother housing eleven people in a two-bedroom apartment at times. We did not have much, and I received NOTHING on a silver platter, everything I had was earned.

During my middle and high school years, my dad *still* chose to be "missing in action" (MIA) and drug-addicted. Unfortunately, my mother battled illicit drug use for a short period during this time also. Actually, I had several family members on drugs. I made a personal vow during my adolescent years that drug-usage would not be a part of *my* story. This part of my personal journey plagued me for some time... at times I *felt* accursed, inadequate, unloved, and somehow destined to be punished for the sins of my father; but I had a loving and praying grandmother! Up until her recent death I always cherished and honored my grandmother; she was the stable consistency that I needed. I know that much of who I am is because of her! Academic excellence was not a toilsome feat; it came very easy for me (I was one of those students). Often due to personal family situations, I intentionally submerged myself in school, friends, and work. I realize now that *this* was a coping mechanism.

I started working at the age of fourteen, I was a bagger and worked my way up to a cashier at a local grocery store. I worked throughout high school and played basketball. I recall many of days not having family in the stands at my games or having a ride from practices. Thankfully my teammates parents or my coach or whoever my grandmother could pay to pick me up got me home. I still played my hardest though and loved the sport. Although I graduated high school a year early, no one encouraged me to go to college. I was advised to graduate high school and get a good job [with benefits]. Looking back, I realize these people could only advise me from the level of perception and success they had for themselves. Fortunately, God gave me the desire to want more. When I graduated from high school my mom *was clean and working* and moved away to another town but I chose to stay in my hometown and finish high school. I really got to see God's power manifested through my mom during this time because not only did he clean her up he also gave her a new start and gave me my best friend back full of faith. What he did in her life made me a believer. My mom had returned to school and became a nurse herself. She purchased a car for me as a graduation gift. I was elated and extremely grateful! The car signified new beginnings for me and the road lead to limitless opportunities; the first being college enrollment.

No one accompanied me to freshman orientation; I applied and registered for college *alone;* however, I was on my way to being *Nurse Te*. During my first year of college I became a mother. I was afraid and uncertain; but I did not relish in the fact that "I was not ready to be a mom" at all. Ironically, during this time God birthed an unstoppable drive within me [I still have this same drive – just stronger]. I refused to allow being a teenage parent to stop me from achieving my personal career goals! I was determined to be a nurse *eventually*. There were days and nights I thought about giving up, but the tenacity God gave me would not allow me to bow out; but instead, it pushed me relentlessly. Having a child made it difficult for me to focus on my studies. Furthermore, the financial demand to provide for my son caused me to alter my plans. Subsequently, I enrolled in a CNA course, so I could work within the field I planned to make a career of. My journey was rough – the constant starting and stopping but I maintained two jobs [at times] and took classes at night.

At one point I was put on academic probation because my grades suffered due to my inability to focus wholeheartedly. My financial aid was revoked and I paid out of pocket until I could get back into satisfactory standing but I had to simply prove to myself that nothing would *stop* me. After working as a CNA for quite some time, I was fired due to lies and the intentional malicious sabotage and envy of a fellow colleague. It saddens me to say that her efforts were successful and I momentarily gave up on my dream of being a nurse. I had never experienced that type of hostility in a work environment; my termination was *almost* relieving!

After being fired I transitioned into customer service as a bank teller and worked my way up to a teller manager. During this time, I was involved in a very unhealthy abusive relationship. I vividly remember an unsuccessful attempt to camouflage my bruises with makeup and one day a coworker spotted the physical shame and abuse on my face and she URGED me to get out! I stayed longer than I should have, but God kept me and allowed me to escape... *alive!* I hid the abuse from my family, I feared the judgment and I was not ready to acknowledge the hurt and shame. However, as my son got older, I reconciled within myself that I would rather be alive and healing from my past versus being a memory *of the past.* Furthermore, I cringed at the thought of my son growing up in an environment where domestic violence "was the norm." I refused to let him grow up thinking abuse was okay (my son would NOT learn and repeat this behavior). When I planned my escape, the abuse had escalated from *bad to nearly fatal...* I literally went into hiding to save our [my son and I] lives.

I remained in customer service for approximately ten years. Then one day I had an epiphany that put me in a state of utter dissatisfaction (I realized, I had allowed complacency to creep into my life). I remember it like it was yesterday. I sat on my bed, staring in disbelief and I felt completely outdone with the circumstances of my life. I was living paycheck to paycheck and I knew I was not fulfilling the purpose of *my* life. At that moment, I decided I was going back to school to attain my LPN license. I called my husband (yes God sent me a good husband) and my mom to inform them of my decision. I didn't know how I would accomplish this. Truth be told we were struggling with two incomes and the program required me to be fully committed; keeping my current job was NOT an option - at all. *This was scary!* This was a real-life faith walk for my husband and me.

In 2005, I resigned from my job and enrolled in the PN program. I will not lie and say this was easy because it was far from it. I experienced days of crying, second guessing my decision, broke and received a lot of harassing phone calls from bill collectors; but I tried to continue to focus on the light at the end of the tunnel and not my current state. I knew I had to do this for my family, especially my sons. We had two boys at this time and I didn't want to preach the importance of getting a college education to them and I not be that example myself. During my low moments, my husband and mom would build me up with the encouragement I needed to finish the race set before me. My goal was to complete the LPN program and work (at a higher rate of pay) while I bridged. I did just that by working through an agency in Corrections and wherever else they would send me. I had a few prerequisites to take before I could apply for the ADN program, but I kept my drive and handled them like a boss. Three years later, I applied and was accepted into the LPN to Bridge to RN program. I went to work at a local hospital on a Medical-Surgical Unit. I was so determined to work and study [tirelessly] and I finished my requirements for an Associate's Degree.

Due to my overwhelming zeal and fortitude, in 2010 I started the BSN program at the University of Central Florida. At the time, my family had grown to a party of five. My husband and I have three boys and my youngest had just started kindergarten. I needed to focus all my attention on my baby boy as he adjusted to school so, I decided to take off one semester and volunteer more at his school; however, that turned into a three-year hiatus. In the meantime, I began to feel like I had learned all I could on the unit I was currently working, so I searched for something more fulfilling. After several bouts of seemingly endless application processes, I was eventually interview and finally landed a job in the Intensive Care Unit. Boy was that scary. I felt like a brand-new nurse all over again but I loved learning this new knowledge and learning to think more critically. Nurse Te had finally found her specialty.

In the summer of 2014, I finally decided to finish what I started and transferred to a local college to obtain my BSN. I was determined to finish this degree even if it meant paying out of pocket. By transferring to a state college, I could obtain my BSN debt free. As far back as I can remember, I have always wanted to be a nurse. Unlike some, my journey to become a ""*Nursepreneur*" did not start early within my professional career. However, this journey has been far from easy but one of the most gratifying accomplishments I have achieved. When I consider my ups and downs and the uncertainty of it all I am grateful for all that God has equipped me to do! I overcame feelings of inadequacy, domestic violence, and teenage parenthood. Every mountain that I have surmounted caused me to realize that God's grace is the *only* reason that I'm *still* standing and able to operate in this capacity!

I have now been a nurse for the last eleven years; and I absolutely love what I do! Unfortunately, while caring for others there was a period in my life when I neglected to give myself the care that I deserved. I tipped the scale at a weight that was much heavier than I desired. The unwanted weight took a toll on my health, and as a nurse the reality of my personal well-being seemed oxymoronic. How could I, Drumeka Rollerson [aka Nurse Te] effectively care for anyone while willfully neglecting to care for myself and *be* the best me possible! Subsequently, my weight loss journey started in 2010.

I utilized the wealth of knowledge I attained from being a nurse and my relative studies. I have lost over thirty pounds and I worked every day to keep it off. Nothing works but WORK. I changed my eating habits and exercised anyway I could and whenever my time permitted [I frequently made time to exercise]. I am still fighting to maintain my weight loss through my lifestyle change. Please understand, this transformation has been one of the hardest things I have ever done, but my determination to reach the goals God *placed inside me*-caused me to feel like "David when he faced Goliath" [What giant? Don't let the cute face fool you]!

As with every shifting in my life, God stretches my faith in Him. During my weight loss journey, I often felt unattractive and unmotivated. I prayed vehemently and asked God to help me move beyond personal insecurities and self-sabotage. I started writing down notes of self-encouragement and I read them faithfully [this was in 2011]! Then God gave me the desire to turn these quotes into a clothing line of fitness attire [in a dream] The line would encourage customers while simultaneously making them feel and look good! I knew my business idea was ingenious because GOD *gave it to me* but... I must be transparent here; I was afraid. I talked myself out of taking this **LEAP**, and I blamed my unwillingness to work this business venture on the busyness of my life and my lack of entrepreneurial knowledge.

Understand this, when God gives us an idea or decides to birth something out of us, there is *nothing* we can do to stop it [although we can delay it – we cannot prevent God's will from being done because IT'S ALREADY ACCOMPLISHED IN HEAVEN]. I gave this preface to illustrate God's grace, favor, and sovereignty. I sat on *Dilan Array* [my fitness attire clothing line, www.dilanarray.com for five years! In September of 2016, *Dilan Array* launched officially, and we are doing phenomenally well! I had some amazing "purpose-pushers" behind this vision. I won't name them in fear of leaving people out; but every customer, website developer, graphic and fashion designer, my husband and family, friends and coworkers helped me see this vision through. I am grateful! My weight loss journey helped me, but it has also helped so many others. Helping others exists at the very core of who I am!

Thankfully, God has allowed me to expand my business ventures in healthcare as well.

Last year in April of 2016, Ocala, Florida officially launched its first and only chapter of Black Nurses Rock (BNR). I am the CEO of BNR Ocala, FL chapter, which was an opportunity granted by none other than God's favor. The sovereignty of God is matchless. The national chapter organizer of Black nRock; trusted me with the local establishment of BNR after a few conversations. Since the establishment of Ocala's BNR, our chapter has exceeded our personal expectations for community outreach local and global healthcare initiatives, and we put Ocala, Florida on the map (just kidding). Seriously, Black Nurses Rock is a non-profit organization with a focus to foster a positive environment of professional growth and development. Locally our mission is to assist driven, determined, and dedicated nurses to grow professionally while addressing healthcare disparities in the Ocala/ Marion county area. We provide support and mentorship to nurses to elevate our profession and improve our communities. Within our first year we were able to give three thousand dollars in nursing scholarships locally. Black Nurses Rock is the largest minority nursing association in the country, representing over 174,000

African American Nurses and students from the USA, Canada, Eastern Caribbean, Africa, Japan, and Germany.

The launching of BNR caused me to go into a state of introspection about a business venture I allowed to lie dormant for too long. Gratefully, on March 25th of this year, *Rollerson Consulting Firm* opened its doors where I am the CEO and primary professional healthcare consultant; *RCF* provides innovative, dedicated, and trustworthy wellness solutions. Since our mobile/virtual doors opened, God has allowed me to witness and experience what happens when we follow his lead and faithfully *work* His will for our lives. There is nothing more gratifying than doing the things you were created to do. I advise anyone who is reading this not to simply be business-minded, but make sure every decision you make is God-centered.

Lastly, I recently jumped into uncharted territory again after many conversations with my business mentor, Dr. Rometrius Moss, and became a radio show host on Hot 104.5; The Nurses Station, launching my own show Health and Fitness Talk with Nurse Te. My show airs Mondays at 5pm EST and my focus is educating on all things health and fitness related so people can live their best lives NOW! I also use this opportunity to help promote other small businesses to get their brands in front of the masses. This is an internet station that is growing daily averaging at about five thousand new listeners a month. Check me out at www.theNursesstation.net on Mondays. I am amazed at what I have accomplished with God when I finally broke up with fear.

There are three things I want [YOU] the readers to remember: (1) Fear is the primary cause of complacency and mediocrity. To achieve YOUR God-ordained greatness, you must not allow fear and uncertainty to paralyze you and keep you stagnantly existing in a place outside of your destiny. In the book of Matthew chapter 14: 26 – 32, Jesus tells his disciples, "Be of good cheer! It is I; do not be afraid…" Like children they still required proof! So, Peter says, "Lord, if it is You, command me to come to You on the water." Jesus said, "Come," and Peter took a step out of the boat without sinking!" Anytime God places a desire in us to do His will (our desires are His will), He will not allow internal circumstances (doubt, fear, uncertainty, feelings of inadequacy) or external circumstances (jobs, people, hardships, or financial woes) to consume us. We will literally walk on water and even if we start to sink, God's grace is sufficient and He will save us from our fears! With faith in Jesus Christ, Peter walked on water. But *when* the strong winds blew, Peter took his focus off Christ and focused on the circumstances surrounding him. Peter's doubts caused him to sink, not his ABILITY to perform the task at hand! As he begins to sink, Peter called for Jesus' help. Jesus immediately stretched out His hand and saved him. As He did so, Jesus asked Peter, "O you of little faith, why did you doubt?" This was a rhetorical question; Jesus knew Peter's faith was shaken so he delivered him! Ironically, even amid Peter's doubt he still walked on water! Case and point… even if you're afraid, still pursue what it is you are seeking to accomplish, do it even if it requires you to ask for help along the way!

Secondly (2): Be purpose driven! Allow your purpose to dictate the direction of your life. Your purpose resides in that nagging, relentless beckoning to do *that* thing or things you dream about, wake up talking about, and irrefutably understand it is what YOUR life is about. Our lives are directly linked to God our Creator-so everything we do is *supposed* to glorify Him- and *make* His name great (not ours)! Our purpose while we are here on this earth is to *do God's will* for our lives. Romans 8:28 states, "And we know that for those who love God all things work together for the good, of those who are called according to His purpose." Therefore, make this declaration from your mouth now, "I will be purpose driven! My purpose is simply to please God in everything that I do (my words, my thoughts, and my deeds)!

Lastly, (3): Surround yourself with like-minded people (even if it's just you – sometimes you will be the *only* person that has the mentality to understand YOUR God-given greatness). Proverbs 13:20 reads, "Whoever walks with the wise becomes wise, but the companion of fools will suffer harm." This is the insight I gathered from this scripture, people who are of like minds inevitably make their peers better. The scripture says "Whoever," thus you may not be the wisest in the group when you surround yourself with go-getters, entrepreneurs, and CEOs, but if you remain with them long enough you will take on the attributes of those people and in turn become the very thing(s) you have admired and studied (wise people study). However, those who become the "Companion" (the friend and confidant) of a fool suffers simply by being associated with them! In other words (unlike the wise), you don't even have to do the things "The Fool" does to experience the harm that follows him; you are affected due to your proximity!

SURROUND YOURSELF WITH LIKE-MINDED PEOPLE... be vigilant, prayerful, and watchful. We know a tree by the fruit it bears. Connect with some Bosses and

Bosstresses.

I will never "toot my own horn," but I will continually strive to achieve greatness! My journey as a Black Entrepreneurial Nurse has been challenging, enlightening, humbling, and empowering all at the same time. Understanding we have an indomitable power within us to accomplish incredible feats will create a space of greatness that *only* we can occupy – please tap into this source. Our source is God – this is an undeniable fact. I desire for every person I meet to be the best version of themselves, I want them to *rock* this thing we call life, and fulfill their God-established purpose as they're doing it! Trust me, I have not just tapped into my Source, but the grip I have is unbreakable. I do NOT just "rock" as a Black Entrepreneurial Nurse, but everything and everyone I encounter has access to the "Rock" because of me! Consequentially, this equates to divine healing, prosperity, health, and wealth. Abundance *is* the portion, and mediocrity has no place among "*Nursepreneurs*" everywhere! I hope and pray my story has inspired, ignited, and invited you to a place of foreseeable greatness. There is nothing more gratifying than excelling in the very things YOU know you were created to do. God is the best event planner you can allow to orchestrate your life… don't allow anyone or anything else to deter you from this fact! Allow HIM to navigate your steps; His plan is for you to prosper and have a phenomenal future. Be blessed and start walking today into your BOSS/BOSSTRESS status. We can all win.

About the Author

Drumeka Rollerson is a Bachelor's prepared Registered Nurse with almost twelve years of experiences in pediatrics, corrections, home health, medical-surgical, and critical care. With interests and passions ranging from community service to educating others on health disparities, Rollerson's mantra of "never giving up and going after your dreams, no matter the obstacles" inspired her to establish a nonprofit organization. As the CEO and Founder of the Ocala's Chapter of Black Nurses Rock, Dilan Array LLC, and Rollerson Consulting Firm, she is a proven and effective leader and mentor. When she is not busy being a wife and mother to three, you can find Rollerson on Hot 104.5, where she fiercely educates her listeners as a host on *The Nurses Station*, which features her *"Health and Fitness Talk with Nurse Te"* show.

To Contact The Author:

Instagram: @Healthandfitnessnursete

@dilanarray

Facebook: Health and Fitness Talk with Nurse Te

Dilan Array

THE NURSEPRAYNEUR: FROM CARE PLANS TO BUSINESS PLANS

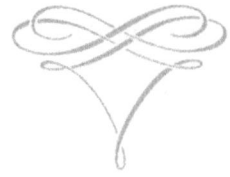

Tamara Alford Neely, Medical Director
NP-C, MSN, BSN, RN, MT

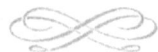

Growing up in a small rural town outside of Raleigh, North Carolina, I knew I wanted a career where I could help others. After graduation from high school, I attended Johnson C. Smith University, an HBCU in Charlotte, North Carolina, on a full scholarship. I majored in biology because of my first mentor, Mr. Hubert Avery. I desired more than "country living and a place where everyone knew you."

After graduating with honors from college, I decided I would attend NC A &T State University to get my Master's in Biology. I knew, during the first week of class, this was not the path for me. Later that year, I decided to become a medical technologist. I worked five years for one of the largest healthcare systems in Charlotte. After working there, I wanted more hands-on care with patients.

I decided to apply to nursing school in 2001. After working as a nurse in a hospital for three years and working just one day with a home care agency in nearby, Gastonia, I decided to start my own business. I worked one day for a non-medical home care agency doing home care assessments. Once the owner told me how successful her business was, a light bulb went off. I would not have to pay someone to be my nursing director; I would be able to save that money, starting out, by not hiring a nurse. Eventually, I could pay a nurse to work part-time as the business grew.

I diligently researched and opened my homecare business

in five months. HomeCare for the Carolinas LLC (HC4C) was born in May 2006. Initially, HC4C serviced low-income individuals receiving Medicaid with non-medical home care services. Later, our agency added Medicaid HIV case management, Ryan White HIV Case Management, and housing for homeless veterans with mental health/substance abuse challenges. After 11.5 years, we continue to make a difference in our clients' lives.

FINDING MY PURPOSE

You must find your purpose in life to really exist and use your God given talents. What is your purpose in life? Have you ever asked why? Why were you born into your family? Why were you born Black, White, Hispanic? Why did you get into an abusive relationship? Why did you have sex with someone you trusted and got an STD/HIV? Why did you get pregnant as a teenager without a husband? What would your life look like without any substance abuse? Why did your business fail? Why did a loved one die? Why did you get divorced? These are some of life's questions that can be the catalyst to starting your own business or finding your purpose. It has been stated that "if you can find out what your passion is, it could be the linkage to your purpose".

I had a desire at a younger age, to help others. While in college at JCSU, I wanted to be a physician's assistant but this never happened. I was not accepted to Duke University in 1994. I did not have the required hands-on experience in healthcare to get accepted. It was a competitive process. After applying twice to Duke University, I didn't have the desire to be a physician's assistant any more. But God had other plans for me! Twenty-two years later, I attended Duke University as a Nurse Practitioner to pursue a post-master's certificate as an HIV specialist! When you serve a mighty God, sometimes He gives you things you never desired.

What is success? Success is not about how much money you make but about how you can change the trajectory of someone else's life. I have been blessed along the way but only through God's grace. Never measure your success against someone else's. This can lead to jealously and envy. I found my passion, my why, and what makes me wake up daily feeling, successful.

It can become easy to compare. Comparison will do two things: First, it can make you feel less than or inferior; or it can make you feel like you are better than or superior. Success does not boast but is humble at all times. You can lose everything that took years to build in a in a blink of an eye. We have all seen celebrities living high then lose material items and show signs of mental instability.

My purpose allowed me to care for my brother. It brought me peace knowing I could spend the last month with my brother when he was placed in Hospice Care for terminal cancer. I was able to be his nurse and show compassion and care with excellence along with my sisters, family, and church family. This was my passion in action. I worked as an unofficial Hospice Nurse; something I never thought I could do. What God allowed was for me to see my purpose at work. You see, your passion or purpose will allow you to transcend/transform and work in other areas of nursing that you did not realize you had the potential to achieve.

WHY DID I WANT TO BE A NURSE ENTREPRENEUR?

I wanted to be a nurse entrepreneur to help and serve those less fortunate and assist in navigating the health care system. I am blessed to learn quickly and help others. I have helped heal and house hundreds of people by doing business for the past 11.5 years. Most of my work has been with the government. This is where I could work with clients from various backgrounds. People often ask me why I want to work with those who have HIV or homeless veterans with mental challenges and substance abuse. The answer is I love what I do, and I would not change anything on my path as a nurse entrepreneur. Along the way, I mastered how to do business with the government. I have worked with (Medicaid, HRSA, VA) to serve the clientele who needed me the most.

MY BUSINESS

I have been in business for 11.5 years. The services we provide are non-medical home care, HIV Case Management, VA Contract housing, and leasing some of our rental properties. We have a very specialized niche where we have been working with the government to help solve some issues clients have, accessing the medical healthcare system. Our services provide cost effective solutions which saves the government money.

We provide non-medical home care where Certified Nursing Aides (CNA) or Personal Care Aides (PCA) go into clients' homes to assist with activities of daily living (ADL) and housekeeping tasks. This program is called Personal Care Services (PCS) in North Carolina. The client gets up to 80 hours per month. Additional hours can be obtained if clients have Dementia, Alzheimer's, or other memory loss conditions. Community Alternative Program (CAP) provides services for clients in their homes. Assistance with ADL's and housekeeping tasks are done by the CNA staff. HIV case management allows the case manager the opportunity to work with the client one-on-one to assist with ambulatory appointments, medications, and medication adherence. Currently, we have two residential group homes which house male veterans in a transitional type of living. We have been working with Veterans Affairs (VA) for the past six years. HC4C also has rental properties which are leased to other companies for passive income.

One of our company's future plans for business is to assist youth by opening a daycare center. I had an in-home daycare licensed by North Carolina in 2001; however, I closed it when I started nursing school. I have always had the desire to help others learn at any age. In addition, we will soon open our spa for massages and facials at our clinic.

MY DEDICATION

I have been blessed to be a blessing to others. I have dedicated my career to assisting others with our services or helping other entrepreneurs start their business. My dedication to the field of nursing has become my ministry. Where else could I make such a profound difference in the lives of people whom I may not have ever met unless I started my own business? I was able to do it on my own terms with my own rules. I am dedicated to the field of healthcare.

10 KEYS TO START A SUCCESSFUL BUSINESS

When you start a business, make sure you start on the right path. I started out small with one service and grew it over the years to have a successful business. Make sure you do not sacrifice your integrity for money. I equate having a successful business to having an honorary MBA. You must put in a lot of work to get established. A successful business is not a get rich quick scheme. Below are 10 keys that will assist you along the way for a successful business.

1. **HIRE YOUR DREAM TEAM.** Hire the right people to work with your team. Make sure you hire people who will run with your vision and have passion for your business. If you hire people who don't align with your vision, this can set your business back years and you may never see success. I have had to fire people who brought too much negativity in the workplace. Remember you can have control of who you choose to hire at your company. Don't be miserable along the journey. Your staff will spend more time with you than some of your family members; therefore, they should be pleasant to work alongside. If you know you lack a certain skill set, you should make sure to hire someone who excels in what you lack.

2. **FIND A MENTOR**. I was blessed to have a mentor in my house growing up as a child. My father, Charles Alford, Sr. is a successful barber in my home town. He opened the first Black barber shop in Benson, North Carolina, when I was in fourth grade. I saw him put in challenging work while working a full-time job. It allowed him to be with family and serve his community. Your mentor needs to have traits of integrity, honesty, and a desire to help others. If you are looking to start a family care home, try to find people in your community who are successful and have operated in business for at least 5-7 years as a family care home. Don't get discouraged if someone does not want to be your mentor or share knowledge with you. Keep trying and ask God to send you a mentor. If you

can't find a mentor, find a peer or hire a coach. Sometimes you will have to invest money in reaching your goals. You can surround yourself with people who are trying to start their own business, by attending local SCORE organizations. SCORE organizations have the largest network of volunteer business mentors who will work with you at no cost. They offer online and in-person workshops.

3. **WORK HARD, PLAY HARDER.** To have a successful business, you need to work HARD. Some people will have to work a full-time job while starting their business or work part-time. The beauty of attaining success is to enjoy the journey. Take time out to enjoy family, friends, and travel. It can be as small as having a pampering day where you go to the movies and out to eat dinner. Make a habit to work out and eat healthy. Give your mind a break by enjoying an hour massage or facial. These are very affordable at beauty schools, Groupon, or Living Social. Some may want to go to the park and see God's nature. These are things that you can enjoy for free if your funds are limited.

4. **NEVER GIVE UP WHEN TIMES ARE HARD**. Put God First and he will carry all your burdens. It is easy to give up on your dreams because it usually requires a lot of work. Sometimes when you want to give up, go volunteer your time with an organization that aligns with the mission and values of your business. If you fall ten times, it is how you get up on the 11th try that counts. Never give up until your last breath. You don't want to look back over your life wondering what if! Remember to try until you succeed. Never give up!

5. **UNDERSTAND YOUR BUSINESS PLAN.** What is a business plan? A business plan should tell us about your company and projections of growth. You can research sample business plans to fit your business. I took a lot of free classes offered on how to write your business plan and was chosen by Small Business Administration as 1 of the 19 inaugural students in Emerging Leaders (Charlotte Chapter). Also, take free classes at the community colleges or throughout the community. Get education on the topic of your interest. Always be willing to learn more for your business.

6. **KEEP IT SIMPLE**. Since we have the internet to research what type of business you would want to start, it can get intimidating when you see the success of others. When you start your business, try to keep it simple by perfecting one type of service. I started out doing non-medical home care first and later added case management then housing. It would have been too much starting out as a new business and hiring staff in this process. As my biology professor would say, K.I.S.S.=Keep it Simply Simple. Even when keeping your business simple, make sure you are strategic with execution.

7. **NO EXCUSES**. When trying to start your business, you may at times come up with a hundred reasons or excuses why now is not the time to start a business. It may be lack of money, education, time, or just self-doubt. It all starts in the mind that you can do it. If you never try, you won't succeed in starting a business. All it takes it faith of a mustard seed. You must step out on faith and put into action plans the birth of your new business. Fear is the biggest reason most never start a business. Don't use fear

as an excuse.

8. **LOVE WHAT YOU DO**. When you love what you do, you are not really working! Try to find a business you can work all night without complaining or you would work for free. Don't start a business that you do not have any interest of keeping long term. Have you ever seen professional athletes leave the game because the desire/love was missing? They left millions of dollars on the table because they would rather be happy than play a sport and be miserable. Always remember to follow your heart!

9. **HAVE THE RIGHT PERSPECTIVE**. Starting your business is like birthing a baby. You need to have a positive experience by surrounding positive people around you. You may have some people saying you should not start a business. You need to know that having this business is an extension of you. You must have the right perspective and don't allow negativity from others abort your dreams or goals of having a successful business. Be confident in all your goals and when you go out in public to represent your business.

10. **USE S.M.A.R.T. GOALS**. If you are a nurse, then you know all about S.M.A.R.T. goals. They should be specific, measurable, achievable, realistic, and time specific. Use this when starting your business. The S.M.A.R.T. goal can be as simple as coming up with your company name as an LLC with a checking account within 30 days. It should be something that you understand and it is your goal and not someone else's goal for you. Remember that we are not trying to keep up with the Jones'. If a goal cannot be measured, it will be hard to track.

HOW TO DO BUSINESS WITH THE GOVERNMENT IN 90 DAYS

I started my business and, after getting my home care license as a non-medical home care business, was able to do work with the government (Medicaid). It took about six weeks to get my provider number for Personal Care Services (PCS) and Community Alternative Program for disabled adults and children (CAP/DA, CAP/C). Working with the government has allowed me to live my life on my own terms. If you want to do business with the government, you must run a legitimate, legal business. Below are 10 steps to start doing business with the government for a contract.

10 Tips to Start Doing Business with the Government

1. Choose a business name and choose which type of business structure will benefit you. This is where you can consult an attorney. You can choose from a sole proprietor, limited liability corporation (LLC), S-Corporation, or C corporation. Corporations protects your personal assets and gives your business a nine-digit tax-ID number. You can go online at https://www.irs-ein-tax-id.com to get your Employer Identification Number (EIN). You can get this number in an email usually within an hour on the same day if done during business hours. As a sole proprietor, all profits and losses are reported on your individual tax return and the entity is not taxed. Also, you will have unlimited liability for your business debt as the only owner. If you decide to do a LLC, you can have can have one or more owners and you must file and register with your

state. In North Carolina, I must file every year and pay $202 electronically. LLCs are liable for investments and protect your personal belongings. A C-corporation requires you to have a board of directors/officers, annual meetings, annual reporting requirements with an unlimited number of shareholders. These are usually large corporations such as Microsoft, Wal-Mart, and Ford. There are double taxation and dividends are taxed at the individual level if given to the shareholder. Lastly, an S-corporation is required to have a board of directors/officers, annual meetings, and annual reporting with an unlimited number of shareholders. S-corps differ from C-corps because the entity is not taxed, and the profit and losses are passed to the shareholders and reported on the individual tax return (Schedule K). Again, talk to an attorney to see which setup for your business is best.

2. Open a bank account. Shop around for a free business account. Make sure you get a folder with a copy of EIN, Articles of Incorporation, Business license, or trade name information. You will need some of this information when opening a bank account. I have free accounts at Wells Fargo Bank and Fifth Third Bank. Do your research.

3. Register your business with Duns and Bradstreet. Duns and Bradstreet gives you a data universal number (D-U-N-S) which is a nine-digit identifier so other lenders and potential business will learn about your business credit or financial stability. You can call 1-866-794-1577 for technical assistance. While free for businesses required to register with the US Federal government for grants

and contracts, they will try to sell other products to you. Also, you can complete online at https://iupdate.dnb.com/iUpdate/companylookup.htm

4. Locate your North American Industry Classification System (NAICES) Code. This is a 6-digit code that classify your industry. Some of the codes that I have used to work with the VA are:

NAICS Code:
623220 -- Residential Mental Health and Substance Abuse Facilities
623990 -- Other Residential Care Facilities

5. Register your business at www.sam.gov. This is something that you can do for free. Make sure you go to the correct website to avoid sites that charge you. Don't use www.sam.com unless you want to pay. You will need to update your business every year at sam.gov. If this is not active, you will not be allowed to do any contracts or receive money from the government.

6. Get the necessary insurance to do government contracts. Shop around for the best insurance for your needs. You may work with an insurance broker to find multiple companies to compare several insurance companies at one time. You will be required to obtain insurance at the time of the contract. The solicitation will tell you the required amounts of insurance to do the contract.

7. Register your business as a HUB-Zone disadvantaged business (HUB Zone) if your business meets the requirement. If you are a minority female business

owner with majority ownership, get your Minority Women Small Business Entity (MWSBE) or Women Owned Small Business (WOSB). There are set-asides for small businesses and the government has a goal of awarding 3% of all dollars for prime government contracts. I have my business as a HUB Zone and WOSB.

8. Research for contracts. Go to https://www.fbo.gov/index

    This site you will need to play around with, so you can become familiar with how to search for contracts. You can search by states, NAICS codes, or agencies. You can do an advanced search form to get specific information on a contract in which you are interested.

9. Attend workshops. Sometimes you can find out if local government entities are having workshops to review upcoming requests for proposals or contracts before the bids are due to be turned in.

10. Apply for a contract if you meet the qualifications. Some may require you to have prior experience. I started doing the VA contracts with limited experience. We have now been doing the VA contracts for the longest in the Charlotte region.

A PRAYER FOR YOUR BUSINESS'S SUCCESS

May God bless us daily with our business to help everyone we meet along our journey. Give each one of us the spirit of courage and faith with perseverance as we make new contacts with the right customers. Please do not let fear exist but a spirit of faith. May our focus always bring joy to you Father God. Bless us with the right staff so we can make an impact on all of those who we will serve.

Thank you, Father God!

Amen

Each of you should use whatever gift you have received to serve others, as faithful stewards of God's grace in its various forms. Peter 4:10

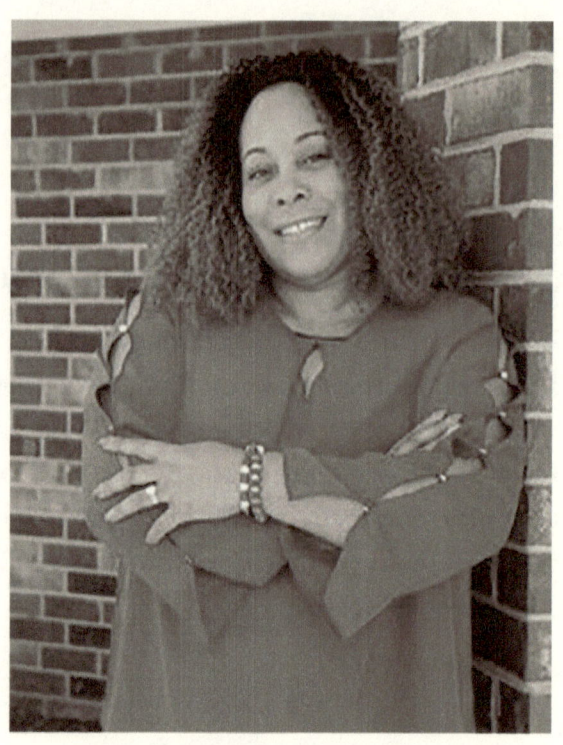

About the Author

Tamara Alford Neely has been the wife of Meredith Neely for 19 years and is mother of teenager, Makayla. She is a Christian who puts God first in her life. She was raised in rural Benson, North Carolina and currently lives in Charlotte, NC. She serves as the Medical Director for her clinic and non-medical home care business. She has been a Nurse Practitioner since 2014. She is an HIV Specialist receiving her training from Duke University. She has been in business for 11.5 years providing non-medical home care services, HIV case management, and housing to male veterans with mental health/substance abuse issues.

Tamara has been a nurse since 2003. She received her training from Carolinas College of Health Sciences, Winston Salem State University, UNC at Charlotte, and Duke University. Currently, she is enrolled at Anderson University to become a Psychiatric Mental Health Nurse Practitioner (PMHNP). Before nursing, Tamara went to JCSU to obtain a BS in Biology and worked as a Medical Technologist in the hospital for five years. Her training was done at Carolinas College of Health Science for Medical Technology to work as a Generalist Lab Technologist.

Tamara started her 501 (c)3, The RISE Project of the Carolinas, in 2008 to start doing government contracts with HRSA. Her first government contract was with Mecklenburg County Health Department doing emergency financial assistances and case management working with the community of minorities who have HIV. She has received many grants/contracts since 2008 and written grants for other companies.

She has opened two family care homes and two multi-family housing facilities with services in Charlotte, NC. She has a real estate company, Neely Realty & Investments, which provides rental property and commercial properties in the Charlotte area. She enjoys teaching others about first time home ownership. She believes in giving back and helping others.

She serves as a mentor and coach for others in the healthcare business. Her company, HC4C, has given out three scholarships for the past two years to assist freshmen going to college. She is a consultant for those wanting to start a business in the healthcare area. Her next venture is to restart a daycare business she once owned in 2001.

To Contact The Author:

Email: tamneely@gmail.com

Facebook: 7 FiGure NursePRAYneur

Linked In: Tamara A Neely

Twitter: @tamaraneely1913

NOT YOUR AVERAGE NURSE

Latosha Annan, MSN, RN, DNS-C, CM/DN

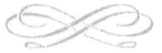

JUST A TYPICAL DAY

The alarm clock rang at 5am on a Tuesday morning. No one else was awake. Lilly laid in bed for a few minutes and then slowly got up to begin her busy day. She headed to the bathroom for a quick shower as she stepped and stumbled over toys and clothes that the kids didn't put away the previous night. She then went downstairs to finish dinner she had started the night before. As she went downstairs she became upset as she found out the dishes hadn't been washed the night before and she refused to cook in a dirty kitchen. By this time, her husband had gotten up from all the noise heard from the kitchen, so he went down to check things out. He saw how busy and upset Lilly was and offered to clean the kitchen and finish cooking dinner. She took him up on his offer and went upstairs to get the baby ready for daycare. At this time, she realized how quickly time was passing and began to panic so she took a few minutes to pray. Praying allowed her to calm down and refocus on the tasks at hand.

Time was ticking and she needed to leave soon to make it to work on time. Before leaving, she left instructions for her husband about making sure the kids ate breakfast, was dressed appropriately and arrived at school on time. She headed out just a few minutes past her normal time. When she got in the car, she turned the Bluetooth on and began doing her morning devotion. Usually, Lilly prays with the family but on days like this, she had to resort to having prayer over the phone. Lilly had overcome the morning routine obstacle but now it was time to face the world as a full-time senior nursing leader and part-time entrepreneur. As soon as she entered the building - even before she could get her bag off her shoulder - the staff immediately hit her with multiple issues at one time. Lilly was a little overwhelmed, but she tackled one issue after another and eventually got things settled down. She finally reached her office to look at her calendar to see what was lined up for the day. With a manager out sick and floor staff short, she knew it would be a long day.

At the end of her 11-hour work day, Lilly realized she hadn't eaten, used the bathroom or even taken a sip of water. She was weak, tired, drained, overwhelmed and just plain emotionally and physically exhausted. On the drive home, she reflected on the day and became sad and disappointed as she thought about the many sports games, recitals, and other performances she had missed because she was stuck at work for eleven to twelve hours a day. She arrived home to the faces of disappointed kids because they had planned to go out to dinner, but at that point, it was too late. The kids had to opt for Ramen Noodles instead. Lilly was angry and disappointed at herself. She never wanted her children to feel the pain of their mother coming home late from work and not keeping dinner plans. After explaining the hectic day she had, Lilly settled down to eat and shower. She had only been asleep for an hour when the phone rang. She looked at her phone and when she saw the number, her heart skipped a few beats. She braced herself for the conversation ahead. On the other end of the receiver, was the nursing supervisor calling to say there were three call outs. The nursing supervisor informed Lilly that she could cover all but one slot. After being at work all day and getting only one hour of sleep, that was the last thing she wanted to hear. Unfortunately, there was no other option; Lilly had to go in to cover the 11pm-7am shift. She angrily got dressed, kissed her husband and kids, and drove back to work. Lilly arrived at work and sat in the car for about ten minutes trying to calm herself down before going inside. Once inside, she called every nurse on the call list, but who in their right mind would pick up the phone. They knew the number and knew exactly why someone from the job would be calling at THAT time. No one responded. Lilly worked for six hours before the next shift staff arrived to relieve her. Being in that situation really opened Lilly's eyes. She never wanted that to happen to her and her family again.

When Lilly arrived home, she was comforted by her family and the breakfast her husband had already prepared for her. As she made her way upstairs, she noticed the dishes were washed and put away, the floor was swept and mopped and all was well. She gave her husband a big hug and kiss with final words of thank you and I love you, as she headed to her awaiting bed. She was so exhausted that she only took a few bites of her breakfast before falling into a deep sleep. Lilly slept over 11 hours.

> The demands put on nurses are not getting any lighter. We are constantly being put in overwhelming situations with very little resources. We are asked to work long hours, with few if any breaks. Often, we work short staffed but are required to provide the same level of care as if we have adequate staffing.
>
> These unreasonable demands lead to burn out. This phenomenon has led many nurses to become an entrepreneur.

OVER THE EDGE

For years, but only in her mind, Lilly pictured herself as a business owner, an entrepreneur, a CEO, a boss. No more clocking in and clocking out, interrupted family dinners, asking permission to take the kids to doctor's appointments, mandatory overtime, or being forced to discipline an employee for something with which she did not agree. As she sat at a red light one day, she began daydreaming and replayed a day when she was having a meeting with her boss. She couldn't help but think about the words spoken to her and they constantly echoed. "As Senior Nurse Leader and maybe one day Nurse Executive..." and "You will only go as far as I will allow you to go." Those words resonated within her soul like nothing before. Her boss was implying that she was the deciding factor in Lilly's future. When she got home she reminded her husband of this incident and after much talking and praying, he gave her his full support and encouragement to step out on faith. Lilly was determined to not let anyone have such control over her destination, except for God of course, but live out her full potential as God - not man - has determined. She went downstairs to the kitchen table and began to map out her plan to be in business for herself. She first explored the many options available to her as a nurse in business such as:

1. Nurse Consultant
2. Personal Care/ Assistant Instructor
3. CPR/First Aid Instructor
4. Delegating Nurse
5. Specific Disease Educator (ex. CHF/COPD, Diabetes)

6. Allied Health Instructor
7. Home Care Agency Owner
8. Staffing Agency Owner
9. Assisted Living Owner
10. Legal Nurse Consultant
11. Health Coach
12. Geriatric Care Manager
13. Health Blogger

> What's your passion? Find your niche. The opportunities are endless!

Lilly wrestled with the idea of becoming an entrepreneur. How would she start? How would she stay the course? This was not her first time at trying her hand at starting a business so she knew to stay on course this time, she would have to focus on what would truly motivate her. Would it be her desire to provide quality care, the need for flexibility, potential for increased income, her family or the opportunity to challenge herself?

Lilly spent the next few months educating herself on various aspects of being a business owner. She felt that anything pertaining to her field of expertise would be easy but everything else that came with entrepreneurship could be a challenge. She often wondered to herself if she really had what it takes to start, run, and grow a business. She questioned if she was ready to take on the added responsibility of not just providing a service but managing all the other components of being an entrepreneur such as accounting/bookkeeping, managing the office, marketing (promoting and pursuing new clients), networking, and serving as client relations manager.

Lilly quickly realized starting a business was not a decision to be taken lightly. She needed to think seriously about whether this was something she was willing to do. Was this another addition to her pocket full of dreams or just a phase she was going through because of the words that were spoken to her by her boss? With everything else on her plate, she had to understand the significant commitment and sacrifice of personal time and energy this venture would entail. She asked herself, "Am I ready, willing, and able to start, run, and grow a consulting business?" After much prayer and waiting on the Lord and with her husband's approval, her answer was YES! But with very little money to work with, three children, and need to have a steady income, how could she start a business? She figured since she was equipped with special knowledge and experience in the field of nursing and had relationships that could be transformed into business opportunities, Lilly was off to great start. Yes, she was correct. However, to sustain a business, her enthusiasm and passion had to extend well beyond mere consulting to starting, running and growing a business as well.

> Develop a comprehensive business plan. If you are not seeking funding, try starting with a lean startup business plan.

When Lilly first started out on the journey, she often times found herself fearful. She frequently thanked God for her husband, who was a Godly man, a leader, a man of prayer. He was always very supportive and encouraging, especially when she felt like giving up. When Lilly would become fearful, her husband would always take her back to the scriptures, reminding her of what God says and not rely on how she felt or how things looked at the time.

GRIPPED WITH FEAR

According to dictionary.com, Fear is a distressing emotion aroused by impending danger, evil, pain, whether the threat is real or imagined.

Although Lilly had financial support from her husband to maintain their way of living, there was no way they could survive on one income. She was at a crossroad... Either stay on the current path or take the road of greatest resistance - entrepreneurship. She was making a decent salary, the job location was not too far from her home, she was familiar with the staff, co-workers, residents and she was able to tackle the daily tasks given to her... why should she change anything? How could she leave what she considered financial security? What if she couldn't get clients? Where would the money come from to buy the necessary items needed to start, run and grow the business? What if something unexpected happened? What if she provided a service and the client didn't pay her? How would the bills at home get paid? Should she get a credit card? And then what if she couldn't afford to pay the money back? How would she make it through the early stages of running a business from a financial perspective? So many questions. Unfortunately, Lilly did not have wealthy family members or friends to ask for money nor did she have $100,000 in the bank or a trust fund from which to pull money. She was faced with the decision to start consulting part-time as she continued to miserably work full-time at her job, or step out on faith and free fall into entrepreneurship. What was she to do? Despite all the opposition and fear she was facing, Lilly took the free fall, knowing her husband would be there to catch her if she fell. He was a man of great faith and would surely cover her through prayer.

> Have consistent presence on social media. Look for opportunities to advertise your business in your local community.

OFF TO A GOOD START

Once Lilly was over the initial feeling of fear of being in the dark, having the car repossessed, not having enough food to eat, getting evicted, and simply being embarrassed to face family, friends, and neighbors - she was just fine. She constantly reminded herself of Matthew 6: 28-30 which says, "And why do you worry about clothes? See how the flowers of the field grow. They do not labor or spin. Yet I tell you that not even Solomon in all his splendor was not dressed like one of these. If that is how God clothes the grass of the field which is here today, and tomorrow is thrown into the fire, will he not much more clothe you—you of little faith?"

Lilly was so enthusiastic and steadfast about working on a business plan, she would wake up early and go to bed late. She had to be sure her business idea solved a problem and that she created a service she would want to use as a consumer herself. She did lots of research, including competitors, initial opportunities, opportunities for growth, weaknesses and threats to her business. As she researched, she identified additional services/products she could offer that was not a part of her original business plan. Identifying these additional services helped Lilly stand out amongst the rest. Over time she realized there were other components she needed consider. How would she market (social media, lawn signs, networking events, word of mouth, radio, television, cold calling, or advertising in the local newspaper)? How would she structure and operate her business? What kind of business entity would she need to set up? Would she need to set up a corporation or LLC? Would she do it herself or hire a consultant to help her? Would she hire employees, either full-time or part-time or would she hire independent contractors? Would she buy or lease an office space and equipment, or start out at home with what she had? Who could she turn to for guidance? While at a conference a few months before, Lilly remembered hearing about the recommendation of getting a business mentor. So, she began searching, but was not successful.

> Make networking and building relationships a priority.

DOUBT

According to dictionary.com To doubt means to be uncertain about; consider questionable or unlikely; hesitate to believe.

The word was spreading that Lilly had started a consulting business and people began asking her why she had left her "good job" for something that may not even work out. One of her close friends even took her out to lunch to explain her point of view as to why her decision to start a consulting business probably was not a good idea. Lilly's friend started their lunch date by listing all the pros to working for someone. Pointing out the fact that as an employee, unless something drastic happened, Lilly knew she would receive a paycheck, taxation was easier, and she would get paid vacation days. She even reminded Lilly of all the other business ventures Lilly tried her hand at but was not successful. The lunch date lasted for about two hours. Later that day, Lilly thought about the conversation when she laid down to rest. She began to question her decision. "Did I make a selfish move?", she thought. Am I jeopardizing the future of my family?, Did I make a bad call? Lilly discussed her encounter with her friend and how she was feeling with her husband. He assured her that he would support her in any way he could; but more importantly, he encouraged her to pray to God for guidance because ultimately, He was in control. Lilly prayed daily about the situation and began to slow her efforts down to wait for an answer from God. Weeks went by and Lilly became very frustrated, overwhelmed, and anxious because she still needed to finalize her business plan. She tried reaching out to other consultants in her field and called entities that would utilize the services she was offering, but she got nowhere. With no one willing to help her, the fear became increasingly intense. After many difficult days filled with "No's" and uncertainty, she decided it would be easier to just go back to being an employee. She thought if the process was this difficult so early in the game, there would be no way she could be successful at starting, running and growing a business.

WEIGHED DOWN BY PROCRASTINATION

According to dictionary.com, Procrastination is defined as putting off or delaying, especially something requiring immediate attention.

Lilly decided to sign up for work with a nursing agency where she could clock in, do her work, and clock out. Simple right! She wouldn't have to worry about client acquisition and retention, marketing, bookkeeping, client relations or anything else. Although she had a different assignment every day, she was back in her comfort zone. Lilly became so complacent with just punching in and out that her desire to being an entrepreneur slowly began to diminish. Talk about De Ja Vu. After about 4 months of working with the agency, she realized that there was a difference between ensuring she had a well thought out plan and paranoia. Of course, she needed to prepare, line all her ducks in a row, dot her I's, and cross her T's; but she could never plan for every single situation that could arise. The most important factor would be her response to those issues. For the next few months, she found herself going back and forth with the idea of continuing to work with the agency or work toward her goal of being an entrepreneur. She found herself growing more and more frustrated and annoyed. Not with the fact that she didn't enjoy what she was doing, but with the limitations of her ability to impact those who she cared for. She eventually found herself moving forward with becoming an entrepreneur and not giving herself any other option. There was no turning back and regardless of the situation; she was determined to never resort to the cousin of fear, who is procrastination again. She couldn't be hindered by what-ifs, maybes, suppose this happens, and suppose that happens. If she allowed herself to stumble over fear, doubt and procrastination, she would never know the opportunities available to her. Initially, Lilly had to maintain her employment at the agency while building the business part-time and still maintaining her status as a wife, mother, nurse, counselor, cook, housekeeper, chauffeur, teacher, etc.

ALL OR NOTHING

She thought about the business plan she had started months before and now understood it was a working document and would evolve over time. Over the past months, even though she had not been actively working on developing the business, Lilly had matured as an entrepreneur. She had been researching and attending seminars, conferences, and webinars. She realized the greatest impact in getting people to know who she was and what she had to offer was through networking. She realized that as an entrepreneur, networking would be the most powerful tool in her toolbox. Lilly joined groups in her local and adjacent communities, on Facebook, Linked In, Twitter, and Instagram. She also continued to attend conferences and seminars related to her area of expertise and learned to always have business cards and/or brochures on hand.

During her time of networking, she built relationships which translated into clients. Eventually, Lilly even expanded the networking concept by making herself available for public speaking. She developed a quick elevator speech about herself as a consultant and the business which she could quickly and comfortably communicate in conversation with new acquaintances.

After researching different business structures, she decided to set up an LLC; and to save money, she did it herself. She officially registered the business, finalized the business logo design and opened a business savings and checking account. She had to cut expenses wherever she could, so she found a website that completed her logo for only $10 and she designed business cards and brochures herself at a reasonable price. Lilly used a spare room in her house as the home office and decided to not hire anyone until she reached a certain number of clients. Lilly had to be creative in letting money work for her, so she negotiated her first contracts by asking for an advance payment for part of the fee or charged a retainer fee. For business sustainability, operating with good character and integrity helped her reputation and allowed her to stand out for excellence, but word of mouth was powerful as well. She always did her best and worked for her clients with an attitude of dedication, service and a passion for quality and excellence. Lilly recognized that excellent skills and a good reputation alone would not keep her in business. Her reputation for competence and integrity among friends and colleagues may have gotten her first clients as she was just starting, but she couldn't expect it to grow drastically without conscious and very intentional marketing and promotional efforts. Lilly understood she needed to continuously expand her network of relationships that could serve as a pipeline for new business. Marketing her business became her passion.

Looking back, the journey came with many sacrifices such as early mornings, late nights, having to meet with clients despite how exhausted she felt, her husband being upset because she was preoccupied with working on things for the business and sometimes going without income for 3-4 weeks. Lilly focused heavily on marketing and building relationships. People had to know the brand, who she was, and the services she could provide. So many opportunities started to come her way that while in one month, her calendar was filled for the upcoming month. Eventually, she had to hire independent contractors to help her with opportunities that presented themselves. Lilly understood that starting a business was difficult but she also realized that it was even more challenging to maintain a business. After being in business for a while, Lilly remembered her journey as an entrepreneur and all the obstacles she had to face. She wanted to make the journey a little easier for aspiring entrepreneurs by sharing all she knew to anyone who wanted to know.

A tagline Lilly was often reminded of when transitioning from employee to entrepreneur was "I was once blind but now I see". Had she not had a supportive husband and gotten over the feelings of fear, doubt, and procrastination, by reminding herself that God has not given her a spirit of fear but of power, love, and sound mind, she would have never been able to experience freedom and independence to this degree. As long as God gave her life and strength, to some extent, she decided what hours she would work, how much she would like to be paid, and when she would take off. She no longer needed permission from "her boss" to take her children to the doctor, take a vacation, come in late so she could attend activities at the kids' school or to leave work early because she was not feeling well.

What about you? What will it take to make you say enough is enough? In the end, Lilly realized that being an entrepreneur is a mindset. She couldn't be motivated by emotions because her emotions - as with all of us - change minute-by-minute, day-by-day. She would have to stay focused and endure the highs, lows, and plateaus of business. Lilly learned everyone's path is different and not cookie cutter. Some aspiring entrepreneurs may be able to leave their full-time job altogether; some can work their full-time job and work their business full-time; some can work their job part-time and work their business part-time. The point is that each person must figure out what will motivate them and what works best for them given their situation. To move forward, Lilly had to be passionate about what she was pursuing and have a strong WHY?

If you are an aspiring entrepreneur, I encourage you to sit down and map out your goals for 1, 3 and 5 years. Create a vision board. Determine what steps you need to take to achieve the goal. How will you track progress? Be sure your goals are specific, measurable, and attainable. Be aggressive but realistic and be sure to attach a time limit as to when you want to achieve each goal. While pursuing your goals, it is common to experience feelings of doubt, fear, and procrastination; but if you combine what you're great at, with what you love, you'll have fulfillment your entire life. Nothing worth having will come easy. If you have been bitten by the entrepreneur bug, explore opportunities and pray that God leads you to do what He has called you to do. We all have a purpose. Walk in YOURS! Always remember to trust in the LORD in all your ways and don't lean on your own understanding but in all your ways acknowledge Him and He will direct your path.

In writing this book, my aim is to encourage anyone who is thinking about becoming their own boss. It's perfectly normal to experience with fear, doubt, procrastination along the way, how you respond to those feelings is what will be the determining factor. Always remember that if anybody has done it before, so can you. Acknowledge God in all you do and He will direct my path. That's a promise! Perseverance and never give up, for Be confident in who you are and what you can do, for it's better to try and fail than to never try at all. Know your worth. Also, if this endeavor is tackled by a couple, both have to share responsibilities to make it work. Both parties have to do their best to support each other. Husbands need to hold the fort down while the wife is taking care of business. He might have to absorb some of the responsibilities of the wife and visa versa.

YOU CAN DO IT!!

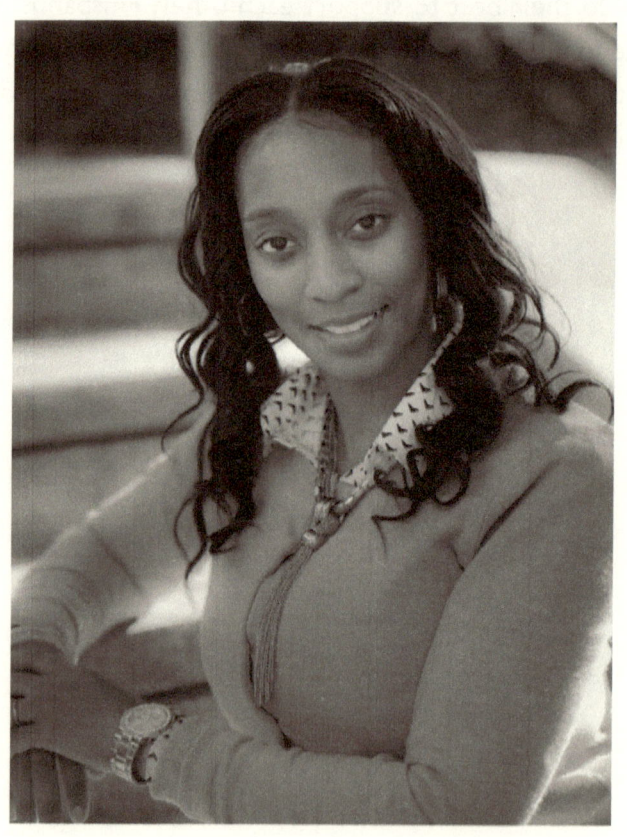

About the Author

A Baltimore native, Latosha Annan is a Master's level prepared nurse with 15 years of experience. She obtained her Bachelor of Science in Nursing from Coppin State University and her Master of Science in Nursing from Towson State University. Having worked in over ten different areas of nursing, Latosha set out to be a well-rounded nurse. Her desire to ensure seniors receive quality care, led her to transition from her senior leadership position to pursue entrepreneurship. When she is not managing the day-to-day activities of her consulting business, she enjoys spending quality time with her family and friends. Latosha is the wife of Felix Annan for 12 years and mom of 3 children, Kirsten, Joshua and Nilah and mentor to aspiring Nurseprenuers. Whenever she finds herself facing obstacles, she reminds herself of her favorite scripture, Jeremiah 32:27 "I am the Lord, the God of all mankind. Is anything too hard for me?" The answer is NO!

To Contact The Author:

Email: qualassuranthealthcare@gmail.com

Website: www.qualassuranthealthcare.com

Facebook: QualAssurant Healthcare Solutions

References:

ADN, B. (2005). Tips for Nurses in their First Year of Nursing. Retrieved from http://allNurses.com/first-year-after/tips-for-Nurses-109924.html

BAYADA Home Health Care. 10 Reasons Home Healthcare is Meaningful Work. Retrieved from http://blog.bayada.com/cares/bid/344231/10-reasons-home-health-care-is-meaningful-work

Carlson, K. (2017). 10 Survival Tips for New Nurses. Retrieved from http://Nurse.org/articles/10-survival-tips-for-new-Nurses/

Entrepreneur. (2017). Senior Home Care Agency. Retrieved from https://onedrive.live.com/edit.aspx?cid=b8ffe6115862bfce&page=view&resid=b8ffe6115862bfce!134&parId=b8ffe6115862bfce!103&app=Word

Franchise Opportunities.com. (n.d.). Senior Care Industry Outlook and Trends. Retrieved from https://www.franchiseopportunities.com/industry-profile/senior-care-industry

Harper, M. (2015). 6 Challenges Most Senior Home Care Companies Face and How to Solve Those. Retrieved from https://www.saviicare.com/blog/6-challenges-most-senior-home-care-companies-face-and-how-to-solve-those

RN Central. (2010). If You Want to Be a Nurse You Better Love to Learn. Retrieved from http://www.rncentral.com/Nursing-library/if_you_want_to_be_a_Nurse_you_better_love_to_learn/

Strebe, S. (2017). You Don't Need a College Degree to Be Successful—Here's Why. Retrieved from http://www.mydomaine.com/why-you-dont-need-a-college-degree

Thomas, L. (2017). Home Caregivers. Retrieved from https://www.senioradvice.com/articles/senior-home-care-registered-Nurses-versus-home-caregivers

Vannuci, M. J. & Weinstein, S. M. (2017). The Nurse Entrepreneur: Empowerment Needs, Challenges, and Self-Care Practices. Retrieved from https://www.dovepress.com/the-Nurse-entrepreneur-empowerment-needs-challenges-and-self-care-prac-peer-reviewed-fulltext-article-NRR

---

[i] Minority Nurse (2015). Nursing Statistics: Get the latest nursing statistics and graphics in the U.S. Retrieved from http://minoritynurse.com/nursing-statistics/.

[ii] Spetz, Joanne (2016). The nursing profession, diversity, and wages. *Health Services Research, 51*(2), 505-510.

[iii] Alexander, Susan (2016). Nurses in business: The time is now. *Clinical Nurse Specialist, 30*(2), 86-88.

[iv] Moore, Jean & Continelli, Tracey (2016). Racial/ethnic pay disparities among Registered Nurses (RNs) in U.S. hospitals: An economic regression decomposition. *Health Services Research, 51*(2), 511-529.

www.ingramcontent.com/pod-product-compliance
Lightning Source LLC
Chambersburg PA
CBHW020650220526
45464CB00001B/370